P A N D O R A   P R E S S

NO TIME
FOR WOMEN

Charmian Kenner spent three years as a health education worker in Fulham, employed by the NHS. She worked with local women's groups and girls' groups discussing health information. She now works in community education running women's health courses. She has also been involved in the Women and Work Hazards group, and in campaigns to improve contraception and abortion facilities. She has one child and lives in South London.

Cover Design by Marion Dalley.

D1075947

NO TIME FOR WOMEN

Exploring women's health
in the 1930s and today

Charmian Kenner

PANDORA PRESS

London, Boston, Melbourne and Henley

First published in 1985
by Pandora Press
(Routledge & Kegan Paul plc)

14 Leicester Square, London WC2H 7PH, England

9 Park Street, Boston, Mass. 02108, USA

464 St Kilda Road, Melbourne,
Victoria 3004, Australia and

Broadway House, Newtown Road,
Henley-on-Thames, Oxon RG9 1EN, England

Photoset in 10 on 11½ Century Schoolbook and Bembo
by Kelly Typesetting Ltd, Bradford-on-Avon, Wiltshire
and printed in Great Britain

Library of Congress Cataloging in Publication Data

Kenner, Charmian, 1954–
No time for women.

Includes index.
1. Women – Health and hygiene. 2. Women – Health
and hygiene – History. 3. Health education of women.
I. Title.
RA564.85.K46   1985   362.1′088042   84–5861
British Library CIP data available

ISBN 0–86358–032–7

This book is dedicated to my mother,
Jill Kenner, with love and admiration.

CONTENTS

ILLUSTRATIONS

ACKNOWLEDGMENTS

The author and publishers would like to thank the following for kind permission to reproduce material in this book: plate 2, Hammersmith and Fulham Public Libraries; plates 3, 11, 13, 15, 18a, 23, Labour Party Library; plates 4, 6, 7, 14, Manchester Studies Archive of Family Photographs, Manchester Polytechnic; plate 6, also Elsie Stringer; plate 14, also Sheila Ingham; plates 5, 9, 17, 25, Gina Glover/Photo Co-op; plates 8, 24, Liz Mackie; plates 10, 18b, Fawcett Library, City of London Polytechnic, and National Association for Maternal and Child Welfare; plates 16 (right-hand side), 20 (original poster), the Health Education Council, London; plate 16 (left-hand side), Peckham Health Group; plate 21, Vivien Seal, and Lambeth Toys; plate 26, Anne Allen.

ABOUT 'NO TIME FOR WOMEN'

Who is this book for?

This book is for all the women who are asking questions about our health – how can we stay well? what causes the illnesses we have? how can we get the kind of health services we want?

Every day women grow stronger and take on more challenges – through parents' groups, women's health courses, women's action groups, or by ourselves. This book contains ideas and information which can help to support us.

From what point of view is this book written?

The basic idea of the book is that we need a society in which everyone has healthy living conditions and good welfare services. At present, many people have neither, and so become ill. We also need a society in which every woman can choose how she wants to lead her own life. At present, we learn only to fit into certain roles, which can cause us stress and illness.

Women, men and children could all be healthier if we lived in a more just and equal society: where every kind of work (including housework and looking after children) was shared out, and where we could all be involved in making decisions according to everyone's needs.

Why does the book use history?

Sometimes it's hard to see our own situation clearly. We are too close to our own lives to be able to stand back and see what is happening. We take things for granted – what our children, husbands, lovers, friends expect of us and what we do for them, what our health problems are and what we decide to do about them.

That is why looking back in history can be very helpful – it's like looking into a pool of water with its surface ruffled by the wind, and then suddenly it's still. You see a clear picture in the water and you realise that it isn't exactly you and yet it isn't totally different. Maybe reflections can tell us a lot about ourselves.

We don't have to look back very far to find a picture of women which is startling and yet very close to us. The women living through the 1920s and 1930s in Britain might be our grand-mothers or our mothers, or in some cases ourselves. They also had to deal with a time of economic depression. We may be shocked by the ill-health women experienced fifty years ago, and by the way in which women often accepted this as their lot – this can make us think *why* it might have been this way, and from there we could start to think about our own health.

We also find that women sometimes stood up for themselves and demanded better lives (why have their stories not been taught to us before?). Today women are campaigning to keep hospitals from being closed, to improve health and safety at work, to be re-housed from decaying tower blocks. In all our struggles, we can draw strength from the women who have gone before us – and their original and inventive forms of action can give us new inspiration.

Why is the book called 'No Time for Women'?

'There seems no time for women, but the men make time,' wrote a woman with five children, in 1914.

Women are brought up to believe that we must always put others first – that other people depend on us to fulfil their physical and emotional needs. We are eternally responsible for keeping things going.

In doing this, we give up our own time, and our own health. 'No time for my own ailments which I have got used to now,' said a woman caring for her sick husband in 1938. We never even have much chance to find out what it would be like to 'be ourselves' or lead our own lives.

It is made out to be 'natural' that women should look after others – as if it follows inevitably from the fact that women bear children. To this one biological fact, all kinds of social expectations have been added. Women are seen as responsible for looking after children, for doing the housework, for working in servicing jobs outside the home, and in general for caring, listening, 'being there' for others. The strain tells on us, causing many problems for our mental and physical health.

We can see this happening to women in other countries and at other times in history: in a Third World village where women do all the household work *and* go out with the herds, carrying their small babies concealed in their shawls – or in Britain in the 1930s, where women struggled to make ends meet with a family on the dole.

There is another sense in which there is 'no time for women'. Amongst the people who seem to have no time for us are many of those in authority, the politicians, employers and officials who work in organisations and agencies which rarely benefit women. They seem to expect us to look after people's health at home for no money at all, or, in jobs outside the home, for very low pay. They do not seem to care if this work makes women exhausted and ill. The welfare services provided for us often do not meet our needs.

And finally, the 1980s is 'no time for women'. Nor were the 1920s and the 1930s. In periods of economic depression, women's burden increases. We are told we have less right to jobs and to pay. Yet work at home doubles – making less money go further, coping with cutbacks in welfare services.

We can rightfully be angry that our health suffers in these ways. Why should there be 'no time for women'?

Learning from women's own words

The book includes many quotations from women themselves. We often begin to think about our situation when we hear that other women have had experiences like ours. We put two and two together and realise that we are not alone – something bigger is going on.

For this reason, I've often used a quotation from one woman, which seems to echo a common feeling, instead of statistics about a thousand women. The statistics certainly exist: the booklist suggests places where you can find more information. But there is not much space in this book, and I decided to use it in the ways that would feel most immediate and personal to women.

It is unusual to make women's words so important. Often, what we know through our lives is put down as 'just your experience'. We are told that the truth only comes through 'hard facts'. But let's be clear that some 'hard facts' are misleading or wrong. When I wanted to find out about women's health fifty years ago, I decided to read women's words first. I read letters written by working-class women to the birth control campaigner, Marie Stopes, telling her of their desperate need for birth control or abortion. I read women's answers to a questionnaire about their health. After that, I read Government reports. I found that often they were not telling the truth – or they were avoiding it. What was written down in many official documents had little to do with women's lives.

The same thing can happen today. We need to question everything we hear – on TV, in the papers, in Parliament. We need to make our own investigations to find out the truth.

How this book can be used

In each chapter, information from history is immediately followed by questions about what happens now – and possible answers. The book contains many pictures, and each of these has a lot to say – they can spark off ideas just as the words can. The idea is to help us look critically at our health problems, the health services, Government policies on welfare, the health information given to us, and women's action. There is one chapter on each of these themes. A women's group could read a particular section together to start off a discussion. You could use the quizzes at the end of the chapters, which ask your opinions on what has been said in the book. With each quiz there are quotations from a group of women, the parents from a playgroup, who answered the questions and discussed them together.

At the end of each chapter there are suggestions for action about health – steps that we might take in a group or by ourselves, to understand more or to try to change something. Chapter 5, especially, is devoted to examples of women's action.

Acknowledgments and thanks

I want to acknowledge all the campaigns and ideas coming from women which are *not* covered in this book. I have tried to write about what I've learnt personally from history, and from women I've met and worked with. I hope most women reading this book will find *some* echoes of their own experience, but many may not find nearly enough. I hope that many other books will be written by different women about health, from their own points of view.

When you're writing you need support from other people. I want to thank *all* those who have given me help and advice (their names would almost fill another book!), including: Jane Black, Juliet Coke, Angie Cotter, Christine Dixon, Maggie Eisner, Judith Emanuel, Wendy Farrant, Pat Gonsalves, Eileen Kelly, Khanum Women's Group (Fulham), Anne Lamming, Jane Lewis, London Feminist Health Education Officers Group, Caroline MacKeith, Sylvia Mills, Munster Park Playgroup (Fulham), Wendy Pengelly, Platt Bridge Women's Group (Wigan), Juneray Raymond, Rochdale Well Woman Clinic, Joanna Roll, Dorothy Sheridan, Julia South, Kathy Tait, Linda Tovey, Jacky Ward, Georgina Webster, Nancy Worcester. Special thanks to Sue Williams for giving me constant encouragement over the years, and helping to write the quizzes and choose the pictures.

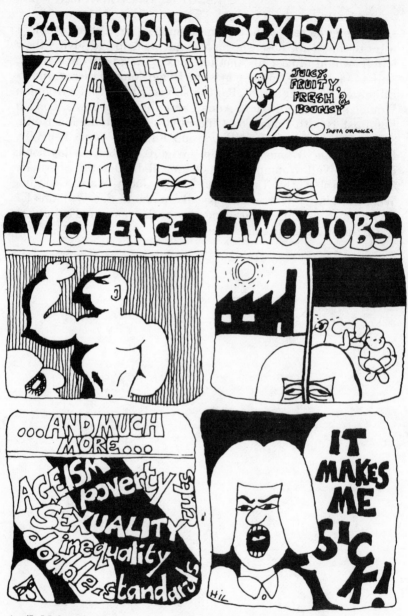

1   'It Makes Me Sick!': cartoon for Women and Health Conference
publicity, 1981
These are just a few of the things which affect our physical and mental
health.

Chapter 1

THE VICIOUS CIRCLE
Women's experience of ill-health

Introduction: The need for a wider approach to women's health

Our state of health reflects our lives. Women's health is determined by the whole of women's lives – by the work we do, the kind of housing we live in, the food we eat, the health care available to us, our relationships with other people.

Our health is not encompassed totally in our biology. The words 'women's health' often bring to mind something to do with our monthly cycles, or with pregnancy and childbirth. Yet women are people with all the rest of our bodies and minds! We have many other health needs which are just as important. Also, when looking at our biology, we cannot separate it out from other aspects of our lives. For example, pregnancy can be a health problem if we can't afford to eat properly, or if we have to do stressful work as well – or if we didn't want a child in the first place. And pre-menstrual tension, although it is obviously connected with our biology, may also be a way of letting out the frustration we feel most of the time.

It is vital to fight for control over what are obviously 'women's questions', such as our experience of childbirth. It is equally vital that we give *all* areas of our health that same close attention. We can then speak out against the *many* ways in which this society damages our bodies and our minds.

This chapter illustrates a broad approach to women's health. By looking at the everyday lives of women in the 1920s and 1930s, and then of women in the 1980s, we can draw out the connections between our experience of ill-health and the circumstances in which we live.

Work outside the home

Working in shops, factories, hospitals, and laundries, women were constantly exhausted and ill. They described their conditions vividly; a woman worker in a lampshade factory in the 1930s reported that:

1

'The girls were expected to do needlework and paint with frozen hands and terrible chilblains . . . the air was often filled with fumes of spirit dye . . . and the girls breathed it in and got coloured nostrils, but they dare not complain for fear of losing their job.'

A woman who *did* lose her job at a Lucas factory in Birmingham, for protesting against speed-up of the production line, said:

'We have to work our guts out, and are speeded up till we get our fingers caught in the drill (and one girl got her hair in and was scalped) . . . no time to blow your nose or go to the toilet. It's a killing job, and I'm glad I'm out of it.'

Protest often meant dismissal. Few women were organised in unions – only 2 per cent of women in engineering were unionised in 1933.

Employers knew that women were particularly vulnerable to exploitation, because paid work had to be combined with looking after the family. They persuaded women to do shiftwork, with the incentive that it would give 'more time' for housework and shopping. When interviewed for a Government inquiry in 1920, many women workers agreed – they could see no other option. They began their day by travelling to work at four in the morning. When they came home, they worked without a break until late at night.

Women's labour was stretched to the limit at times of unemployment. Although only 10 per cent of married women had paid work according to the 1931 census, many were working in that twilight area of 'unofficial' jobs: cleaning, taking in laundry, doing early morning newspaper rounds, bringing needlework home from the factory: 'I can't get out to work so I take in sewing to do and very often don't get paid for my work as I ought to.' As a man who grew up in the North East in the 1930s said: 'It was baking one day, washing the next day, sewing the next day, and hookey mats the next day. That was my old mother's life.'

Women's paid work had the same problems as housework: long hours of standing, repetitive tasks, airlessness, and bad feeding – all disastrous for health.

• What are women's working conditions like now?

Often we are not aware that our work causes health problems – until it is too late. Yet shiftwork in factories and hospitals is stressful and can lead to ulcers. Hairdressing and kitchen work can both involve chemicals which cause dermatitis. Women who work in operating theatres may have miscarriages due to anaesthetic gases. New technology brings new hazards: for example, women stare at visual display units for seven hours a day, getting headaches and bad eyesight.

Employers often treat black women with the least concern; many face working conditions similar to those of the 1930s. Asian women working in an engineering factory said in 1980:

> 'The metal dust gets all over my face, my lips are coated with it and my eyes smart.'

> 'I had to clean out the machine shavings from the oil using my bare hands. I developed rashes and swellings all over my body.'

> 'To speed up production our tea breaks have been reduced to eight minutes. If you want to go to the toilet at another time you are told "do it in your sari".' (information from Black Workers' Support Group)

● Doesn't the Health and Safety at Work Act help women?

This Act is supposed to make sure that workplaces are safe; many employers take little notice of it. Union safety representatives can push for changes, but it takes anger, confidence and organisation to protest. Women are used to accepting their conditions – at home or in a paid job.

> 'It's not really satisfying or dissatisfying.'

> 'It's a good job, because at least it's clean here.' (women factory workers)

Many women dare not speak out if they are not in a union, for fear of being victimised.

Finally, union work takes time – something women rarely have.

● Is it easier for women to combine work and home?

Half of all married women now go out to work, and many women who are single parents have a very hard struggle to make ends meet. Women often do shiftwork so that they can fit in housework and childcare as well, or take in work to do at home – sewing, toy-making – tiring work for tiny amounts of money. Childminding all day and cleaning at night, two jobs, three jobs, four jobs, more jobs. . . . Women work desperately to survive, at the expense of their health.

Housing and household work

Women with families spent most of their time at home, so they were greatly affected by housing problems.

The Women's Health Enquiry, published in 1939, investigated the lives of 1,250 working-class women. Only 7 per cent of them were in 'good' housing (often on isolated new estates). One-third of the women lived in 'intolerable' conditions – housing full of vermin, with water and sanitation elsewhere:

> *'the house we pay nine shillings for will blow you from one end to the other it is not fit for pigs to keep warm in.'*

> *'I have tried for eight or nine years to get a fresh house but cannot get one when you say you have children.'*

Women battled with dust and dirt, breathed damp stale air, carried heavy loads of water and coal, and got an hour's fresh air a day if they were lucky. Seventeen-hour days of heavy housework were common: 'Have no wash-house, and coal-house is downstairs; clothes are boiled on kitchen fire, stairs are very tiring.' If people in the household were on shiftwork, this created a continual round of meals and cleaning up, from dawn to midnight. The job was endless. In better housing, standards rose: 'I work and work all day and cannot see what I have done.'

Standing led to varicose veins and swollen legs, lifting to backache, damp conditions to rheumatism and arthritis, lack of toilets to constipation, crowded rooms to mental stress. Women gave their own examples, such as:

> *'bad hearing for four years, the living room is the cause which causes a terrible lot of steam and dampness.'*

> *'I began to get Bad Headache and this I think is really being shut up in such a small flat with such a large family and when all the Doors are shut, it is so dark and depressing that is what makes your nerves bad.'*

Feeling ultimately responsible for the household was physically and emotionally exhausting, particularly in times of unemployment. One woman described 'sinking feeling in stomach during unemployment period', another 'severe headaches . . . worry due to my husband's unemployment and slack times and how to make ends meet'.

There *was* no time for women: 'I don't get five minutes to myself from morning to night I cry hour after hour to think what I go through lately.' Leisure usually meant other kinds of work. As a woman with eight children put it: 'Leisure time is very scarce as children make work for all time: I take half an hour after dinner to rest and sew.' A real holiday was something which most women achieved perhaps once or twice in a lifetime: 'I really think mothers should have a holiday once a year, I have had one spell of ten days in sixteen years.'

Holidays usually came only when women were ill enough to be considered – by themselves and others – to merit special treatment (perhaps to go to a holiday home by the sea):

> *'I used to feel I was just a machine, until I had my first breakdown, and as dark as it was and as hard as it was it gave me the freedom and privilege of having an hour's fresh air.'*

● Are women's lives at home more comfortable now?

Many slums have gone, yet housing without bathrooms – but with rats and damp – remains. Although many people today live in better physical conditions than in the 1930s, the isolation of high-rise flats can be terrifying:

> *'Someone said that 80% of the women on my estate are on tranquillisers. I'm on the eighth floor it really frightens me. There's no way out once you're in there. It's just square – the rooms are square. If it's a house you can put the baby out in the yard.'*

There is no Health and Safety at Work Act for the home: women are exposed to hazards such as cleaning fluids which can cause skin disease, or asbestos on the work-overalls men bring home to be washed.

● Have labour-saving devices made women's working day shorter?

Women in Britain still do an average of seventy hours' housework a week. Washing machines mean the children can demand clean clothes every day. Vacuum cleaners mean the house *could* be spotless the whole time: 'I think you worry about if someone comes . . . that they're going to walk in and think, oh, *she* doesn't care.'

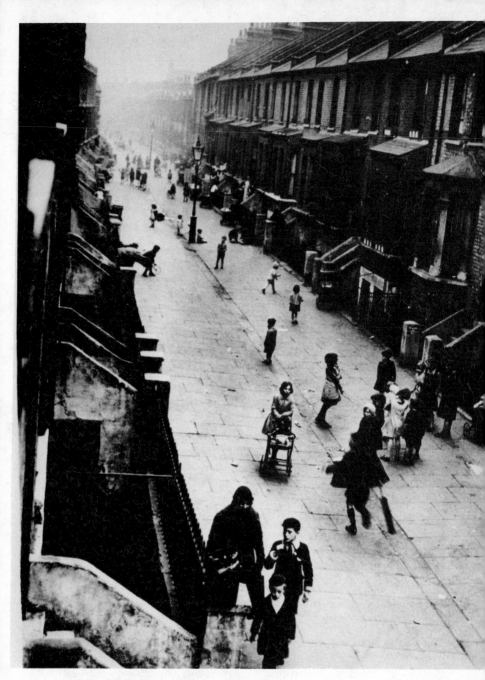

2 Heckfield Place, Fulham, 2 May 1931

Although the houses were probably in bad condition, a street like this had advantages. Children could play safely. Women could talk to neighbours whilst each stood at her front door – see the right-hand side of the street. (Note that there was a pram outside almost every house – many women probably had new babies.)

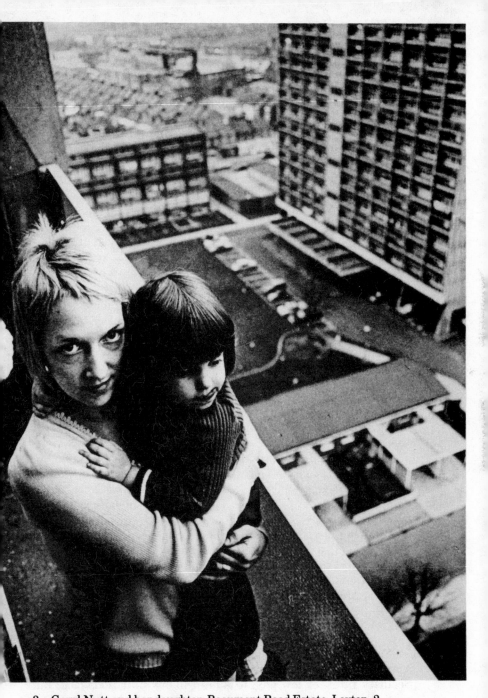

3   Carol Nutt and her daughter, Beaumont Road Estate, Leyton, 2
February 1973
Living in modern tower blocks, women can feel very isolated. You rarely
meet neighbours and there is nowhere safe for children to play. What kind
of housing is best for our health?

Women don't feel they have the right to relax: 'I never really do sit down . . . if I know something has to be done, I'd rather get stuck into it.' Someone else *might* need something.

Thus women's health still suffers because of housing and housework – varicose veins come from standing, bronchitis comes from damp. Headaches, migraine, agoraphobia (fear of going outside) – all can be caused by the anxiety which women feel about their situation.

Food

Food was scarce enough for working–class families. Women had a particularly poor diet, because the habit of self-sacrifice was deeply ingrained – they fed their children and husbands before they fed them-selves: 'Many a time I have had bread and dripping for my dinner, before my husband came home, and said I had my dinner, as I would not wait.' Milk provided by Welfare Centres for women was usually given to the rest of the family. A project to improve women's nutrition in South Wales distributed cans of food labelled 'For Mothers Only'.

Again, time was a problem. Whilst serving the meal and feeding infants, women might only manage a tablespoon of food themselves; as one woman put it bluntly: 'no time for dinner on Monday'. Often women's appetites were small in any case, because of exhaustion and lack of fresh air.

Bad diet and irregular meals led to anaemia, constipation and fatigue. A welfare visitor said of one woman who existed mostly on tea, toast and marge: 'I sometimes wonder to see Mrs. D. alive at all, her children range from 19 to 4½ and as far as I can see she never rests or eats.'

This was a vicious circle in which sickness bred further sickness. Lacking food, women had less resistance to infections. And when a woman fell ill and especially needed better food, nobody else could take over and stretch the budget. Some women did not even feel able to set aside valuable time to teach their children to help them.

● Do women feed themselves better now?

Many people cannot afford to eat properly at present. On Social Security rates, or low pay, it is hard to buy nutritious food. But even when there *is* enough food, some women don't feel they have

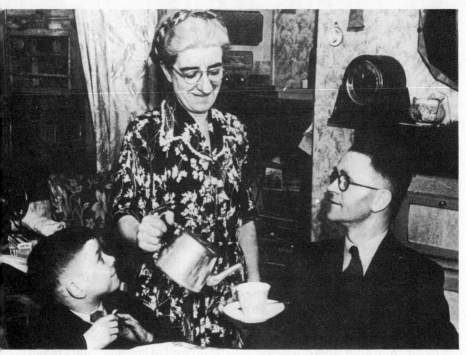

4   Mrs Ross pouring tea for her family, Manchester, 1930s

5   Jackie feeding her children, London, 1980
Feeding the family has always taken up a lot of time. When do women
themselves have the chance to sit down and eat a proper meal?

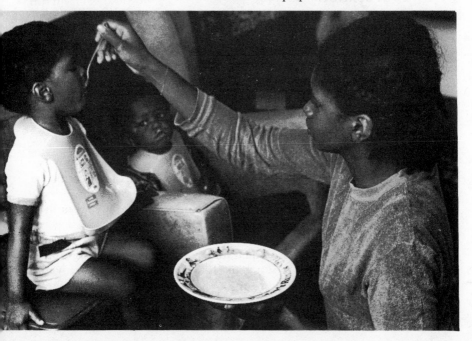

time to eat: 'I just sort of make a drink of tea and a sandwich and I keep going while I'm eating because if I sit down I don't feel like working.' Meanwhile, women are busy feeding the family: 'A fifth of mothers with school-age children don't bother to eat breakfast, but most make sure their children have one.' (*Daily Mirror*, 7 Feb. 1979)

How many women in Britain still give their man more red meat because 'he needs it'? Women's bodies are thought to need less. Yet because of periods, pregnancy, breastfeeding – and hard work! – women actually need *plenty* of protein, iron, calcium and vitamins. 'In Europe, 0% of men are anaemic. 10–25% of women are.' (1976 Unicef Fact Sheet)

Advertising encourages women to eat even less – to become 'slim and attractive'. Women on diets often feel so tense that they start eating biscuits and cakes for comfort, ending up with guilt *and* bad nutrition.

Some women reach for food when they are depressed. Others lose their appetite, especially if they have to eat alone: 'I'll make a meal for my child and by that time I'm sick of the sight of food. And I won't sit there and eat all by myself. One mouthful, that's enough.'

Birth control

Contraceptive knowledge was extremely hard to come by, especially for working-class women. Birth control was not provided at State clinics until 1931, and then only on a very limited basis.

So 'thousands of worn and wretchedly over-burdened mothers' came to voluntary clinics set up by Marie Stopes and others from the early 1920s onwards. They were usually prescribed the cervical cap, used with a jelly or greasy pessary. Other methods included the sponge with quinine or olive oil or vinegar, the condom, and the Dutch cap (more commonly used now).

Problems arose when some husbands were outraged at their wives using birth control. Also, women would have found the cap or sponge inconvenient; they often did not have water in the house to wash the device afterwards. Most women grew up knowing little about their bodies, so putting a cap inside themselves could be embarrassing and difficult.

The sheath was used quite often, but this depended on men's co-operation: 'I have to watch my husband very closely or he would deceive me and not put it on.' Withdrawal was a very common method – and many women avoided sex completely: 'The two occasions (in seven years) on which our two children were created, was when we both consented.'

Women lived with nightmare fears about pregnancy: 'If I had any more children it would most likely cost me my life.' One woman related:

> '[The confinement] was so terrible that only once since then have I allowed my husband sexual relations and then . . . I got up early the next morning and walked fourteen miles in a snowstorm absolutely distracted.'

Another said: 'I suppose many women besides myself will regret Christmas and be waiting for their next period.'

___

• Have birth control methods improved?

There still seems to be no simple, safe method of contraception. Should a woman 'choose' to risk painful periods and pelvic infections (with the coil), or migraine, depression and thrombosis (with the Pill), or heavy bleeding and bad leg pains (with the newest technology on offer, the contraceptive injection)? Are we encouraged to accept side-effects as unavoidable, part of the burden we carry as women? Researchers are looking again at old methods like the cap and the sponge – but to use these we need to feel comfortable about our bodies.

Abortion

___

Abortion was only available to women with serious medical conditions, as decided by a doctor. Yet it was a practical necessity for almost all women. One of Marie Stopes's travelling clinics had eighty requests for abortion in one day – and only thirteen for birth control. Stopes received twenty thousand letters asking for abortion over a period of three months in 1925. Here is one such letter, from her book, *Mother England: A Contemporary History, Self-Written by Those who have had No Historian.*

> 'I am a young woman who has experienced life in every way and have had a very hard struggle. . . . I also am the mother of two very delicate children . . . the doctor just told me the other day that my husband would not live long as he is far gone in consumption. . . . I am not two months

yet and I think it is a greater sin for me to allow this to go on than it would be to try and get rid of it as soon as possible what do you think doctor . . . will you be kind enough to let me know by return . . . it is worrying me ill everyday.'

In her introduction to the book, Stopes said she had cut out 'sentences too intense for publication'.

Clinics could not legally help, so women had to abort themselves. They obtained expensive drugs ('Triumph tablets', 'something for the nerves') from shops or advertisements, often being led on to try 'stronger', equally useless varieties if the first had no effect: 'I took, at intervals, nineteen female pills and a bottle of medicine before I became poorly.'

Lead plasters, alcohol, quinine, herbs, and slippery elm bark, might induce abortion. Chemicals worked by poisoning the woman's whole system: for example, a lead compound called diachylon could cause paralysis and partial blindness. Many women used drugs routinely – 'Although my husband is careful . . . yet I feel tempted every month to take pills' – even after every occasion of intercourse, thus wearing down their health continually.

Women also used syringes and fluid, knitting needles, or tubes of glass or rubber, to perform an abortion on themselves, in their own kitchen, perhaps with the help of a neighbour, sister or mother. 'Each time My husband came home . . . I became Pregnant, and each time I miscarried through my own hand.' Many sought illegal help from a doctor or a local abortionist, who used the same methods. The fee was anything from 2/6d to 3 guineas (whilst a typical wage was £2 or £3 a week). One woman remembered being told 'go to Daisy Hill and take ten shillings there's a woman who'll put you right.'

Some abortionists had midwifery knowledge, or basic experience. Some were respected in the community and earned the gratitude of many women. But complications could arise from not using sterile instruments, or not removing all the contents of the womb, or because women did not have a chance to rest afterwards. Many women died from infection, haemorrhage or shock. Complications following abortions included painful periods, sterility, miscarriage, and haemorrhage in labour.

Women were trapped, condemned to run terrible risks. As one person said of women she knew who were weak from the use of abortion methods:

'They'd rather be like that than have another. And they won't go to the doctor because they say "The doctor'll give me a strengthening medicine

. . . and then I'll fall again." Even after a miss, they manage by themselves, for fear the doctor'll put them right.'

Some women were forced to seek medical help. Many gynaecological beds in hospitals were occupied by women with septic abortions.

• Do women still suffer due to back-street abortions?

Back-street abortion was common in Britain until very recently – abortion only became legal in 1967. For women in many other countries (including Spain and the Republic of Ireland) illegal abortion is still a fact of life. In Chile

'backstreet abortionists use rubber tubes, sticks, barbed wire, vegetable roots and injections. . . . Scores of women arrive every day in the hospitals, with haemorrhages, critically ill. The majority of them belong to the poorest sectors of society.' (a Chilean midwife)

What would happen in Britain if the law was to be made harsher again?

Pregnancy and childbirth

Working-class women faced pregnancy and childbirth under traumatic conditions. Many went through large numbers of pregnancies: to take a few examples from the Women's Health Enquiry –

Mrs. W. of Durham; age 39, 9 children, and one stillbirth
Mrs. T. of Rotherham; 41, 10 children (3 died), 3 stillbirths
Mrs. S. of East London; 31, 3 children (1 died), 4 miscarriages

Unhealthy working conditions were a danger to the woman's body *and* the developing foetus – both could suffer because of poisonous chemicals, fatigue, and bad nutrition. In many workplaces pregnancy automatically meant dismissal – women would try desperately to conceal it, or to get an abortion. By law, women were supposed to stay off work for four weeks after childbirth, but, with no paid maternity leave, 'the old timers gave birth to a child one day and the next few days they were back to work, no grants in those days and convalescence was unheard of'.

Meanwhile, during pregnancy and afterwards, women did not rest from housework. Heavy housework could cause miscarriage: in one case by a washtub slipping and 'causing the child to wedge in some way'.

Some local authorities provided free milk or meals for pregnant and nursing mothers, but women often could not find time to claim this. If there was a charge, a woman thought the money too much to spend on herself: 'Put a penny to it and she could feed the family'. During pregnancy, when they most needed good food, women denied themselves still further, trying to put a little money by for the coming child.

Women who were malnourished had less resistance to infections following childbirth, such as puerperal sepsis, which could kill. A woman who had rickets in childhood might have a badly formed pelvis, making the birth difficult and dangerous. Anaemia could cause general weakness, including weakness in the muscles of the womb, so that labour was long and exhausting. And finally: 'I cannot afford to get the nourishment that I need after a confinement and each one leaves me weaker than ever.'

As the confinement approached, women's anxieties increased: 'I get no sleep and break down many a time because I wonder will the child be all right in brain and limb also I suffer agonies at birth.' Medical services often presented extra dangers: 'I had terrible times . . . having to have instruments and chloroform and the dear little mites cut about.'

About three thousand women died every year in England and Wales, from childbearing or conditions associated with it. If the woman survived, her health would probably have suffered. One doctor estimated that 10 per cent of women giving birth each year were more or less crippled. This was twenty times the number of women who actually died.

Serious prolapse ('dropped womb') was one legacy of childbirth: 'I really no business to have any more as my stomach as got so weak.' Other women commented:

> 'I suffered agonies with womb trouble . . . when it was born I was nearly used up.'

> 'With each child I have found my nerves and eyesight getting worse.'

> 'I am not the same since having she, as I am one mass of sores off and on.'

Breastfeeding was also traumatic under these conditions. Women whose diet did not contain extra calcium might find that their teeth fell out: 'I am hardly fit to go about myself with keeping baby on the breast she is taking all the nourishment out of my body.'

Finally, babies often died: 'the agony of a poor mother when she realises it has all been in vain.' Many were sickly, creating further distress and strain for the woman:

'Last January my oldest girl after ten weeks of suffering passed away at the age of 3½. in Sept. my baby 2 years and 3 months started with Gastric Enteritis and Convulsions and in ten Hours time she also had passed away.'

The onset of menopause, with such a history of ill-health, must often have been difficult – although, ironically, it had its benefits as a release from pregnancy. One woman said of her contemporaries, 'I've heard them say they don't care if they do grow old, so long as the change comes.'

● Do women now have an easier time working during pregnancy?

Many women cannot afford to stop paid work during pregnancy. Hazardous jobs may affect pregnant women even more. A factory worker said: 'This machine involves kicking very hard with one foot. . . . I developed acute stomach pains. Pregnant women had to work on this machine, one of these women had a miscarriage.' (information from Black Workers' Support Group)

Being on your feet all day, carrying small children home up flights of stairs when the lift breaks down – these things can exhaust pregnant women, and cause physical and mental stress.

● Are women well nourished during pregnancy?

A survey in Leeds showed that, in the first three months of pregnancy, substantial numbers of women in all social classes had diets short in energy, vitamins, minerals, or all three, if assessed by reference to the Department of Health's recommended intake for women outside pregnancy.

This could be because women deny themselves food, or can't afford to eat well. Or because the foods widely available to us are bad for our health (see Chapter 3).

● Do pregnancy and childbirth still take their toll of women's health?

Malnourished women who are pregnant are more likely to have toxaemia, a condition which can be fatal. This has been found to be true for women living in poverty, whether in Asia – or in the USA.

New medical technology is not always helpful to women in childbirth. Ironically, procedures like foetal monitoring seem sometimes to make births more difficult (see Chapter 2).

Post-natal depression is common but still rarely talked about: 'It took me over . . . my world became the size of my baby.' Is this a new problem – or has it only recently come out into the open?

Sexuality

Women writing to Marie Stopes often hinted that they could not enjoy their sexuality: the idea of sex could be terrifying, since it usually meant the risk of pregnancy. Many men seem to have insisted on their 'right' to sexual intercourse, even if another pregnancy might be fatal to the woman.

Arguments often arose when women refused sex: 'my husband is getting fed up think how hard it is in one room'; 'it only means living a cat and dog life for both of us'.

Some women seem to have been physically forced into having sex:

'I felt my health giving way, and being in a weak condition, I became an easy prey to sexual intercourse.'

'I simply dread to see night time coming however tired I am because I am always dreading my husband wanting his wishes fulfilled and I am powerless to prevent him.'

Part of the pressure upon women was the deeply ingrained belief that male sexual urges could not be controlled. Women therefore felt guilty for saying 'No':

'My husband has been very considerate, but he cannot deny himself any longer.'

'I feel I am making my husband's life a burden because I have got so nervous.'

'My Husband . . . is a fine big healthy man, but I am wondering if it will eventually injure his health.'

'He had waited patiently for ten months because I was ill. . . . . I submitted as a duty.'

Women were economically as well as emotionally dependent on men. A husband could threaten to go to another woman, or he could refuse to give his wife housekeeping money unless she gave in to his demands. One woman said that refusal of sex 'always makes a man look elsewhere, and I think I would rather have all the children in the world than that'.

Although one woman, in a letter to Marie Stopes, mentioned her own sexual frustration – 'I am very passionate as well as He' – other women did not refer to their sexual needs. Perhaps these needs were simply not aroused, let alone satisfied, by what sex traditionally involved: a man 'wanting his wishes fulfilled' as quickly as possible, rather than the expression of warmth and closeness between two people. As one woman wrote: 'We must let the men know we are human being with ideals, and aspire to something higher than to be mere objects on which they can satisfy themselves.' Another looked forward to the day when 'the man realises that the wife's body belongs to herself'.

● **Do women enjoy sex more now?**

Has there been a 'sexual revolution' since the Pill became available? For many women sex is still a duty. More birth control can simply mean more sex for men.

'Sex? . . . after fifteen years of marriage I still wonder what all the fuss is about.' (a 35-year-old woman)

'I find myself thinking "oh I do wish he'd hurry up." ' (a 16-year-old woman)

Often a woman thinks she is the only one to feel dissatisfied: 'He'd say "you're frigid". He had me believing it, he said it that much. Maybe there *is* something wrong with me, I mean, you never hear other women talking.' Feeling 'used' in sex undermines women's health. With no chance to find out her own sexual desires, a woman may feel completely out of touch with her body.

Women often feel that they have a very different attitude to sex from that of their male partner: as one woman said with amazement, 'After sex he gets straight up and switches on the video.' Many women would like sex to include more emotion and closeness: 'I want affection, touching each other. I want my whole body to be touched and stroked.'

We are taught that sex means intercourse: other ways of making love, such as hugging and kissing, touching and stroking all over our bodies, are called 'petting' or 'foreplay' and seen as inferior. Surveys on sexuality have found that many women (two-thirds or more, according to the *Hite Report*) never have orgasms through intercourse – hardly surprising, since a woman will usually only have a climax if her clitoris is touched, which often does not happen through intercourse.

Knowledge of female sexuality is still kept from us: 'I'd never seen what a woman looked like down there until someone played a joke on my husband and left a pornographic photo in his newspaper.' Many of us therefore grow up without knowing that the clitoris (a small knob of tissue close to the vagina) is the most sensitive place sexually for women.

Because of the view that sex means intercourse, many women cannot imagine how a woman can make love with another woman. Today lesbians are speaking out more openly to express a totally different view of sexuality. But women who were lesbians fifty years ago would have found it even harder to speak out. Why have lesbians always been silenced, insulted, or seen as dangerous?

Women's feelings about their own health

Women felt that they could not *afford* to recognise their ill-health; they must carry on, because they were responsible for the survival of their families: 'Nothing to complain of got to be done so just get on with it and do whatever there is to be done.' Many would have agreed with the woman who said she was well 'in the sense that one is not laid up, and is able to carry on the work cheerfully'. A woman confined to bed would continue to direct household matters, even doing the sewing and ironing herself.

Women measured their health according to very low standards. In answer to questions in the Women's Health Enquiry, many women replied 'yes' to the question 'do you usually feel fit and well?' In answer to the next question, 'what ailments do you suffer from?' the same women listed a whole series of problems, including anaemia, head-aches, constipation, rheumatism, prolapse of the womb, bad teeth and varicose veins.

Over and over again, they excused themselves for speaking of

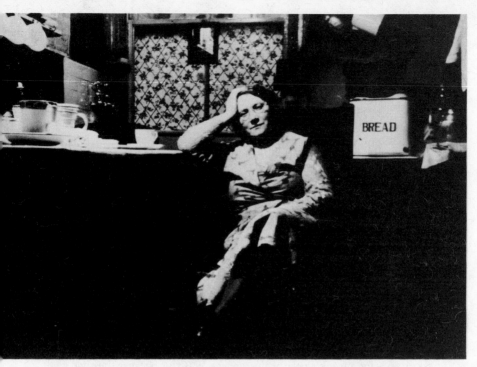

6   Mrs A. V. Jones of Trafford Park, Manchester, in her kitchen, 1934
Mrs Jones's daughter, Elsie Stringer, writes: 'as a child coming home from
school I never remember a day when mother was out. She was always there
. . . a couple of afternoons per week my aunt used to visit for a cup of tea and
they both would be laughing and singing and playing the paper comb . . .
they told each other fortunes in the tea leaves.' Was a tea break most
women's only chance for a rest?

hernia or aching legs as 'a complaint'. Women accepted ill-health as an
inevitable part of their role as mothers, and 'we know some of us have
got to have little children if no one had children the nation would soon
come to an end'. A woman with four children who experienced backache and varicose veins wrote to Marie Stopes, 'I will tell you a little
about myself so you won't think I want it [birth control] from a selfish
point of view.' Harrowing letters to the Women's Co-operative Guild
finished, 'I hope I have not tired you through my letter' or 'I hope this
communication will not offend in any way.'

- ## What health problems do women have today?

There is a lot of chronic (long-term) illness amongst women. In
1978 *Woman's Own* asked readers to answer a questionnaire about

their health problems. The magazine was 'overwhelmed' with replies – listing headaches, depression, heart palpitations, indigestion, rheumatic pains, cystitis. . . .

A recent survey of women factory workers showed that half the women felt continual tiredness. One-third suffered from nervousness, depression, difficulty sleeping, headaches, high blood pressure, sore throats, aching joints, backache, and eyesight problems. Periods caused stress for 40 per cent of the women interviewed.

● Do women value their health more now?

Women still seem to put the family first – and their own health last: 'I never say when I'm ill. . . . I just go on the same . . . it's not worth it, they expect you to keep on trucking anyway.'

Distressing problems are suffered for a long time: 'so after I'd been bleeding for a month I went to the doctor'.

7   Alice Powell and relatives on Blackpool beach, 1920s
Women would recover quickly from most health problems if they had the chance for a week or two at the seaside. Was this because they had a mental break as well as rest and fresh air?

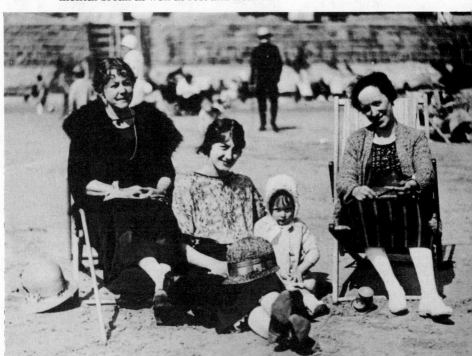

Family relationships and women's health

Low expectations of health fitted with the way women saw life in general. There was a revealing pattern in remarks made about husbands: 'my husband is very good to me *but* . . .' For example: 'my husband is easeful . . . and always willing to help' (compared with the situation she often saw where, with 'women similarly placed . . . their husbands throw their dinner in the fire').

Most men obviously took it for granted that their wives would devote themselves to the home. One woman said:

> *'We do not want to be neglecting the home but . . . if we go to the Clinic we can just have a few minutes. . . . It isn't the men are unkind. It is the old idea we should always be at home.'*

Some men expected work under all circumstances: 'he is rather exacting and has no sympathy with my state of health unless I am actually confined to bed.' Margaret Bondfield of the Labour Party quoted, with irony, a trade unionist who stood up at a conference to say 'Why do we waste time discussing domestic service – we workers never have domestic service – we can't afford it!'

Unemployed men do not seem to have given much help in the house either, perhaps feeling that this would be the final admission of failure, to take on 'women's work'. Thus while men stood, idle and disconsolate, in the street, women remained, harassed and over-worked, in the kitchen.

• Do women get help at home from the rest of the family?

Women often expect (and get) little help from husbands and children. And they still use low standards to measure this help. One woman said in an interview that her husband 'shared the cooking'. It turned out that he made tea and toast on Sunday mornings. 'Well, it's one more cup of tea than my dad ever made my mum,' she commented.

It is unusual for men to help even if they are unemployed: 'The men sit slumped all day . . . smoking endlessly . . . eyes glued to the TV set. To the overburdened wife, it is like having another child constantly around her feet.' (Glasgow GP, 1981)

And the final responsibility always rests with the woman. Her mind is never free: 'No-one else will remember to buy the hamster food, or care whether a six-year-old misses a dentist's appointment.'

Women's health is worn down by working for others. A recent survey showed that married men are healthier than single men . . . but married women are not as healthy as single women. Marriage is a soft option for men – but a tough one for women:

'Miss Jeanetta Thomas, who attributed her health to "non-drinking, non-smoking and the fact that I never married, which meant I had only myself to look after" died at the age of 112 . . . she was the oldest known living person in Britain.' (Guardian, 7 Jan. 1982)

Single women bringing up children alone do not have a man to look after, but often put even more energy into their children: 'You want to make sure your kids don't miss out on anything, you try to give them extra attention, you give them things and go without yourself.'

Violence against women

Many women experienced physical and mental cruelty from their husbands. A woman whose husband was beating her would have had no escape. One woman wrote to Marie Stopes about her daughter's situation:

'he is very ready in useing his hands to her . . . the sheriff told her she would have to go back to her husband or loose her baby as the husband got full controll of her . . . the night before her last baby was born he would not allow her to go to bed she had either to walk the floor or sit in a chair . . . he is always worse to her whenever he knows she is pregnant.'

• How does violence affect women's health now?

It is now publicly known that many women are battered and raped by men at home. Women who left home to go to a Women's Aid refuge said:

'I got kicked unconscious every time. If I'd stayed with him I'd have ended up in a mental hospital. I was cracking up, just cracking up.'

'It's nice to be away from that constant fear. When he used to turn that key – phew, my stomach. . . .'

'Thank God for Women's Aid. I would have left sooner if I'd known about it.'

We know that women feel the constant threat of violence and rape on the street also: 'You can't walk alone round our flats at night, it's terrible.'

Black women, on top of all this, are harassed and terrorised by racism: an Asian woman and her children died in London recently; their home burnt down after a fire-bomb was thrown through the letter-box.

Thus some women receive physical violence. *All* women suffer mentally from living in fear. There is no safe place for women.

Mental health

Many women coped with extraordinary difficulties without – apparently – breaking down, although severe mental strain was often mentioned. For example: 'I was nervous and hysterical: when I walked along the streets I felt that the houses were falling on top of me'; 'Can we any longer wonder why so many married working women are in the lunatic asylums today?' and

> *'The constant struggle with poverty this last four years has made me feel very nervy and irritable . . . when I am especially worried about anything I feel as if I have been engaged in some terrific physical struggle and go utterly limp and for some time unable to move or even think coherently.'*

If a woman *did* fail in her task of keeping the family, the last resort was the workhouse. Unmarried mothers, social outcasts, were especially likely to be sent there. Today there are still women confined in mental hospitals who were put away as unmarried mothers decades ago.

● **How do women cope with mental stress today?**

It is common for women to feel under great strain, from money worries, from looking after husbands who are alcoholic, from anxieties about children's safety. Depression is more often mentioned by women today. Is this because we have more time to think about our situation? Do women sometimes keep busy to *avoid* thinking? Perhaps depression has become an acceptable problem

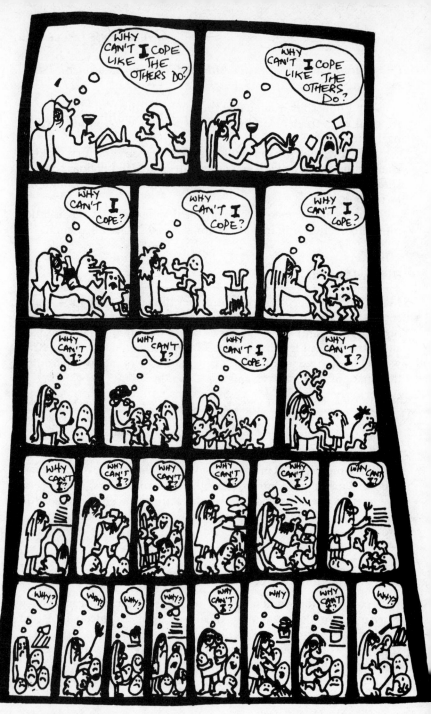

8 'Why Can't *I* Cope?': cartoon
Is this how many women feel? What stops us from talking openly to friends about our problems?

to have. But that is just the point – it is 'accepted' that women are depressed. No action is taken to help!

Some women turn to food, drink or smoking to ease tension – or take tranquillisers: over ten million tranquillisers are taken every day by women in the UK.

For some their situation spells violence: 'The men take it out on us, and we take it out on the kids – but we're the ones that get caught for it!'

There are few communities left where women can seek support down the road – especially if they've moved to a new tower block, or have come to Britain from another country. But often women don't dare to admit difficulties even to friends. Each person struggles on, afraid that she is the only one who is failing to cope: 'I can ask for help but I'm still nervous . . . because it is *my* work. And I feel guilty if I can't manage.'

As a woman factory worker with a family to look after said: 'I suppose you can make yourself a martyr, and you shouldn't do really, should you . . . but I think this all builds up inside you till you explode.'

What would happen if women *did* explode – angrily, demanding positive changes? This chapter has shown that a vicious circle goes on – women are exhausted, ill and depressed, and when you feel that way, you don't have the energy to rebel. We have been brought up to think that life must be like this.

But things could be different – the extraordinary thing is that, despite everything, not all women accepted their lot in the past. And more and more are protesting today. More details in Chapter 5!

Quiz

Try a health quiz – for yourself, with friends. . . . Here are some questions which a group of women answered, with some of the ideas that came up. All the women have young children: we met whilst the children were at a playgroup in the next room. Before doing the quiz, we'd talked about the Women's Health Enquiry of 1938, which showed how tough women's lives used to be.

1 Do you usually feel fit and well?

(a) yes   (b) no   (c) sometimes

Most people said (a), nobody said (b), one or two said (c).

2 Do you have any particular health problems, for example

(a) bad legs   (b) period pains
(c) thrush or cystitis   (d) headaches
(e) anything else?

Each of these affected someone in the group. Other problems mentioned were 'I get tired a lot' (everyone agreed), being overweight, and being depressed.

Do we sometimes 'forget' these ailments, or simply take it for granted that we have them, and still think of ourselves as fit?

'With most women now it seems depression's the worst thing.'

'Well the reason I get depressed, I get bored in the evenings – I've done all the ironing.'

'Yes I never stay in, I'm always out if I can.'

Why did women not mention depression in the past?

'I suppose they wouldn't have had much time to think about it. They might not even have had the word "depression" in those days.'

3 How much time do you spend on your feet most days?

(a) 15 hours   (b) 10 hours

(c) 5 hours   (d) less

Most women answered (a) or (b).

'When I thought about it, it was a lot.'

'All day and night.'

'Well you really are most of the time, because you're watching the children.'

'It's not till you sit down that you realise.'

Before we did the quiz, we'd agreed that it was shocking that women used to be on their feet so much.

4 What activities do you do that you enjoy?

Several women answered 'sleeping'.

'I used to feel like death warmed up in the morning.'

'I've never got up after seven for the last two years . . . they wake up in the night and everything.'

Other people wrote cooking, having a bath, watching TV, taking the children out . . . basic home- and family-centred activities. One person said tennis – and one person said sex.

'You give up your leisure time just to keep going.'

'I do sewing, but that's necessity.'

'Reading is the thing that goes by the board.'

'As soon as I sit down to read I go to sleep.'

'You can't concentrate. You have several things on your mind at once.'

'I have to read escapist fiction – a meaty book I can't get into, you have to find things that can be interrupted.'

What about holidays?

'Well I haven't been on holiday for about ten years.'

'I haven't either.'

This surprised other women in the group.

5 You're dishing out the main course at Sunday dinner. Do you

(a) give everyone the same (except babies and small children)

(b) give your husband more than yourself

(c) give your kids more than yourself

(d) miss out some parts of the meal yourself?

Most people said (a) and a couple said (b). But for a special pudding 'you serve everyone else and give yourself what's left' – and second helpings 'wait and see what's left'.

6 You haven't felt well all day. When it comes to making dinner do you

   (a) still make it

   (b) ask someone else to make it

   (c) go to bed and ask someone to bring you your dinner?

Almost everyone said (a); (c) was thought to be almost a joke – if you were ill enough to go to bed, you'd be much too ill to want any dinner.

> *'I think I've only gone to bed since I was married about twice, because of high blood pressure when I was having Nicky . . . and I've been married ten years.'*

Could husbands be asked to help if you felt ill? Most women said no.

> *'Only if I was in a hot sweat and I looked bad.'*

> *'He'd go up McDonalds, but he'd have to be under extreme pressure, that I'm not putting it on or anything like that.'*

7 Good health is important to women because

   (a) they can enjoy their lives more if they're healthy

   (b) it helps them to cope

   (c) they need to be fit to look after their family

Everyone said (a) *and* (b). Just a few answered (c) as well.

It's encouraging that women can say we deserve to enjoy . ourselves! But most of life seems to be spent trying to cope, and there isn't usually much time left for enjoyment.

This quiz brought out some common health problems for women – especially constant tiredness and anxiety. We also discussed whether other people could help at home, and this part of the discussion is included in Chapter 5, 'How things might be changed'.

Suggested action

For information on how to set up or join a women's group, examples of what such groups have done, organisations to contact for help, and a booklist, see Chapter 5 and final pages.

The following ideas have been used by women's groups to look at health issues:

1 Ask your mother, aunt, grandmother, about the details of her daily life. What kind of work did she do (paid work, household chores, bringing up children)? What health problems did she have? Was she ever depressed and anxious? Does she think women's lives are better now?

2 Make a checklist of health problems (headaches, pre-menstrual tension, not sleeping properly, bad back) and find out how many of them you or the women in your group have. You could also do this at your workplace. Discuss why you think you have these problems – the conditions of your workplace? stress at home? bad housing? lack of health care?

3 Chart your typical day – from morning to night (and through the night!). How many hours do you spend on your feet? Do you have any time to yourself – to do something you enjoy?

4 Consider how you could make time for yourself – by letting other things go for a bit? by asking someone else to do something for *you*? Could you sit down with others in your household and share the housework jobs out? (maybe on a rota basis?) If you start to share responsibilities you may feel that other people don't do the work as carefully as you, but time to yourself could be more important than a perfectly tidy house.

5 Consider what you will do if you can arrange time for yourself. Free time can seem frightening at first, when you are used to always being occupied. What do you enjoy doing? When did you last . . . go out with a friend? have a peaceful bath? read a book? have a conversation which wasn't about children? find out about groups which meet locally?

6 Think whether it's a long time since you last went on holiday. If you want to go away without the children, can someone else look after them just for a couple of days? (Note: women's holiday centres often have cheap rates for women on Social Security – see adverts in *Spare Rib* magazine, address in 'Joining a women's group' section.)

7 Write down everything you ate yesterday – food and drink. Are you feeding yourself regularly, with nourishing food? Are you losing out on food for yourself because you are busy with the children and/or work? Do you find it hard to eat alone? Can you sometimes eat with friends, taking it in turns to cook for one another?

8 Consider how often you need a drink, a cigarette or pills to get by. What stresses cause you to need them? Can anything be done about those stresses?

9 Ask older women about back-street abortions in their community – these stories may never be told otherwise. Talk in a group or with friends about experiences of different birth control methods, abortion, and pregnancy and childbirth today.

10 Discuss how you first learnt about sex. When your first period started, did you know what it was? How would you tell *your* children about sexuality?

11 Draw the outline of a person (life-size) on a sheet of paper on the wall. Mark the areas where it's OK to touch – first, if it's someone you don't know, then, if it's your child, a parent, a woman friend, a man friend, someone with whom you have a sexual relationship. . . . Who can you be affectionate with? Do you get enough affection?

12 Think what you've enjoyed about any sexual experiences you have had – and what you didn't like. What do you think you *might* enjoy? Can you have an equal say about your own needs in a sexual relationship?

13 Try to find out how common domestic violence used to be (local
   libraries have copies of old newspapers which sometimes
   report this) – and how common it is now. How did women cope
   years ago? Do you have a local Women's Aid refuge?

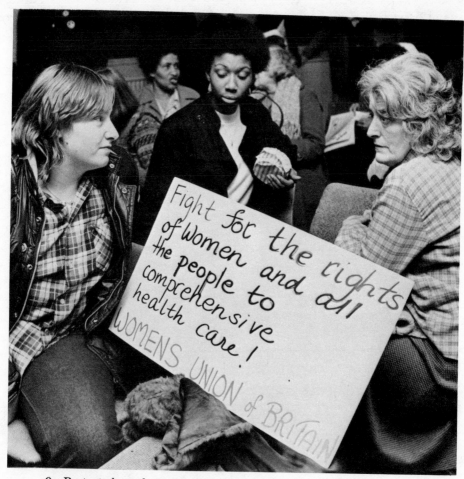

9 Protest about the proposal to close the South London Hospital for
Women, 27 January 1983
These women have met to state that the National Health Service should
continue to provide facilities such as the South London Hospital. Why are
our health services being cut back rather than being improved and
extended?

Chapter 2

HEALTH SERVICES
For mothers only?

Introduction: Women's health is undervalued

Amongst women, many of us undervalue our own health. But people in authority seem to value our health even less. One of their main concerns is that we should have babies, and we often see our children going into factories and wars which profit the powerful.

In the history of the health services, women's own health needs have gone largely unconsidered. Facilities have been directed towards the job we are expected to perform – bearing children and bringing them up. Why do we have many ante-natal clinics and baby clinics, but far fewer well-woman clinics, which should deal with women's general health? Why are women often treated unsympathetically when using the services provided for mothers?

And when we are sick it is often said to be 'natural'. We are told we must suffer 'female complaints' in silence. Sometimes we are even told that we are malingering, pretending to be ill. To avoid recognising that women's ill-health is partly produced by our living and working conditions, those in authority use excuses. They blame our biology, not our society. We need to set the record straight, and campaign for the kind of health services women want.

Women's illnesses – not important?

In the 1920s and 1930s, statistics showed that women and men had different kinds of illnesses. Women were off sick from work because of anaemia, genito-urinary complaints, 'debility' and neuralgia, and many other chronic (long-term) illnesses. Men often suffered from injuries and accidents, and pneumonia, for example. These figures probably showed the effects of work and environment: men's acute (sudden) illnesses were often caused by dangerous work in heavy industry.

Women's conditions – such as bad diet, exhaustion, and nervous strain – slowly wore them down.

Yet men's and women's illnesses were valued differently by the authorities. Men's health problems were seen to be more dramatic and interesting. In 1933, George Newman (Medical Officer at the Ministry of Health) commented that one could observe 'the usual differences' in illness statistics for men and for women that year, 'owing to the greater exposure of men to stress and risk'. He automatically considered women's lives to be less stressful!

As for the risk which most women ran constantly – that of pregnancy – it had been pointed out in 1924 by Dora Russell and other birth control campaigners that *maternity was four times more dangerous than working down a mine*, which was then the most dangerous occupation engaged in by men.

Living and dying

In 1931 men's life expectancy at birth was 58.7 years. Women's was 62.9 years. Yet statistics about *death* ('mortality') told little about the quality of *life*. Statistics on 'morbidity' (health problems during people's lives) were often not collected, especially for women. Health information came from schools, army medicals, and National Health Insurance records. Women who worked at home were invisible in these statistics: their illnesses remained hidden from public view.

• Is women's health adequately investigated now?

Often women are classified by their husband's occupation, so it's hard to find out how women's illnesses are linked to their work. Sometimes women aren't included in health research at all. It is assumed that they are not at risk because they are 'only housewives'. An American study on heart disease simply stated that women are less likely to get heart problems because housework is less stressful than men's jobs: 'the effects are clearly less pernicious'.

The impression is given that executive men suffer most in this society, but working-class men *and* women have a higher rate of heart disease and of many other illnesses. As for anaemia, varicose veins, and gynaecological troubles, these do not receive the same attention as heart disease and lung cancer – yet they ruin women's lives.

Ill-health – the disappearing trick

George Newman reported each year on the health of the nation for the Ministry of Health. His conclusions were always optimistic, even when he had received many reports from local Medical Officers of Health saying that people were suffering from malnutrition, and sometimes from starvation, in the depression of 1931–3.

Perhaps, if his reports had shown a true picture of ill-health, the implication would have been that wide-scale changes in society were needed. Instead, in July 1933, at the height of the depression, the Minister of Health stated to Parliament that 'there is at present no available evidence of any general increase in physical impairment, sickness, or mortality as a result of the economic depression or unemployment.' This was contrary to information from doctors, scientists, public health specialists, and local government officials.

Low standards for women's health

In 1931, when Newman heard that Newcastle Dispensary had an unusually large number of anaemic women patients, he stated that anaemia was 'more closely associated with sickness, pregnancy, postconfinement, lactation etc.' than with unemployment and malnutrition.

So women were expected to be ill because of their biology, and the economic depression was not to be blamed for it!

Newman then said there was not 'any excess in malnutrition or incapacity in women'. (What did he mean by 'excess'?) He finished thus: 'The women in every depressed area . . . are bearing an unusual strain of disappointment and anxiety, but happily there is but little increase of sickness or incapacity directly attributable to it.' In other words, women could be counted upon to cope with all difficulties, and the consequences for their health were of little importance to the Government.

• Is ill-health officially recognised now?

In 1981, Dr Len Fagin finished a report (for the Government) on unemployment and health. He showed that unemployed people and their families suffered from depression, headaches, asthma, constant 'flu, drinking problems, and violence from men towards women and children. Only two hundred copies of this report were printed. Each copy cost £6. The report was given almost no publicity. The Government gave similar treatment to the 1980 Black Report, which showed that working-class people are in much worse health than richer people, and that inequalities in health are *growing*.

Also in 1981, Sir George Young of the Department of Health stated that Government ministers were 'deeply concerned' about the effects of unemployment on health. However, he said, 'We judge that the long-term benefit [of the Government's economic strategy] will more than counter-balance any short-term damage, including any damage to health.'

What is meant by 'short-term damage'? – alcoholism? malnutrition? depression?

Women and health insurance

The National Health Service was not set up until 1948. In the 1920s and 1930s, some women in paid work had health insurance. But insurance societies considered women to be a bad investment.

In 1931, a Government report revealed that insured women claimed more often than men, thus cutting into the societies' profits. Such a situation had been predicted when the Health Insurance Bill was drawn up in 1911: it was said that women were likely to be off work frequently for short-term illnesses. Accordingly, the Bill stated that benefit would not be paid for the first three days of an illness. Also, the pay-out of benefit discriminated against women: women paid 8/9 of the male contribution and received only 4/5 of men's benefit (single women) or 3/4 (married women, who were expected to be dependent on their husbands).

So the authorities *were* aware that women suffered many illnesses. (Women were probably also off work when children were sick.) But insurance schemes, whether private or State-run, intended to make a profit; women's needs came second. A Royal Commission on National Health Insurance in 1926 said that sickness benefit should *not* be extended to women at home, since the costs would be 'prohibitive'.

As for pregnancy, this was the last straw for insurance societies, since it could prove expensive. Some societies refused to pay benefit to women who were off work because of 'a complication of pregnancy', which could mean *any* illness occurring whilst a woman was pregnant, or for several weeks after the birth.

In this way, many of women's health needs were made out to be 'natural' and biological, not the responsibility of society. The 1926 Royal Commission discussed the suggestion to give paid maternity leave. They decided that this should not be done, in case women who worked full-time at home began to ask for money too – and 'such a demand would be peculiarly difficult to resist'. It was obviously better that women's expectations be kept low!

Women as 'malingerers'

Women were said to give 'subjective' evidence about their health, and to be 'suggestible' with regard to illness. When a woman claimed sickness benefit, sick visitors (who were sometimes men – supposedly 'objective'?) were often sent to find out if she was still capable of doing housework. If they found her doing any household task, they could disqualify her from benefit.

Of course women, even when ill, had to keep the family going. The Departmental Committee on Malingering (1914–16) heard of the woman who was scrubbing the floor when the visitor arrived, and jumped into bed with her clothes and boots still on – the suspicious official flung back the bedclothes and declared her 'fit for work'.

As a final insult, some societies suspended women from benefit – on grounds of misconduct – if they were found to be suffering from syphilis, almost certainly caught from their husbands!

• Are women now treated equally in the sickness benefit system?

One group of women is still suspected of 'malingering' – disabled married women. In order to receive a 'Housewives' Non-Contributory Invalidity Pension', they have to prove that they are incapable of 'normal household duties'. Recently, many women answered an Equal Opportunities Commission survey about their experiences. One woman wrote: 'They expect you to be both incapable of shuffling around and completely mentally retarded. Unfortunately I am only crippled with rheumatoid arthritis.'

The National Health Service is being cut back, and the Government is encouraging the growth of private medicine. With private insurance schemes, women could be back to the hardships they faced before the NHS: no cover for pregnancy or childbirth, nor for chronic sickness.

Women — childbearers for the Race

Women who paid National Health Insurance via their work could go free to a 'panel doctor' and receive free medicines. But 90 per cent of married women worked entirely at home; they were not covered by National Insurance. Their only free health care (apart from the hated Poor Law Infirmary) was at the maternity and child welfare clinic – and a woman could only go there when pregnant or nursing. The introduction to the Women's Health Enquiry Report (1939) commented: 'the woman comes onto the map of the public conscience only when she is performing the bodily function of producing a child'.

The official idea was that the fitter British mothers were, the fitter British babies – and thus the British race – would be. Women were expected to bring up their children to be workers for industry, and soldiers to win wars and colonise the 'wide spaces of the earth'. One supporter of these 'eugenic' beliefs wrote: 'Those people and nations will no doubt endure who possess the most healthy, intelligent, true-hearted married mothers.' Eugenic views often had similarities to Hitler's ideas in Nazi Germany.

Politicians made saccharine-sweet speeches glorifying the 'mothers of Britain'. But their cynical approach to women occasionally showed through. Sir Robert McCarrison said in a speech to the British Medical Association in 1937:

> 'As well might we regard the taking of a steep hill as a feature additional to the normal function of a motor car as regard the making of a seven pound baby as a feature additional to the normal function of a woman.'

He was supporting the idea of ante-natal care, but his words made women sound like child-bearing machinery which needed servicing.

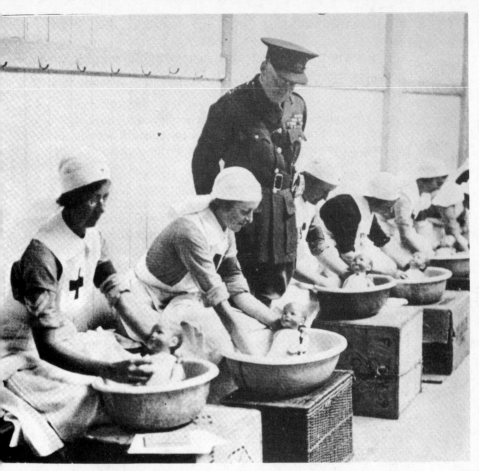

10   General Sir Walter Kirke inspecting a practical class in infant care at
the National V.A.D. Camp, *c.* 1937.
Why was the work of these women being inspected by a man – and by a
man who was a general in the army?

● **How is women's own health valued now?**

In 1976 a woman worker at a Canadian battery-making factory
was told: 'If you want to keep your job, get yourself sterilised.' She
did so. The reason? Lead fumes released in battery-making can
cause miscarriages and stillbirths. The company did not want to
risk being sued if a pregnancy went wrong.

Women are pushed out of hazardous jobs, supposedly to
protect the health of their babies. But what about the effects of the
jobs on women themselves?

- **Are women still encouraged to have babies for the nation?**

A French Government leaflet on pregnancy, produced in 1977, began:

> 'To the mother-to-be: the greatest happiness life has to offer is to be yours. You will take your place in the chain that has no ending of women who are responsible for the continuity of mankind.'

The British Government recently directed health education workers – yet again – to persuade women to attend ante-natal clinics, on the grounds that this was expected to produce healthier babies. Vast amounts of health education literature are produced about pregnancy and childcare; in comparison, little attention is given to other aspects of women's health.

Health services – for women as mothers

From 1918 onwards, the State provided clinics for maternity and child welfare: to look after children's health. Ante-natal clinics, which provided treatment for women themselves, came a poor second. In 1918 there were 2,324 infant welfare clinics, and by 1938, 3,580. In contrast, there were only 120 ante-natal clinics in 1918, and by 1933, still only 1,417.

Not until the 1930s did local authorities begin to provide clinics for general gynaecological care. Clinics for pregnant women were not supposed to attend to these 'other needs'. As for birth control, the Ministry of Health claimed it was 'foreign to the purpose of maternity and child welfare'. Finally, in 1931, the Ministry issued a circular saying that contraception could be given to expectant and nursing mothers if 'medically indicated', but only at a separate clinic session so as not to 'damage the proper work of the Centres'. By 1934, birth control information could be given to women with non-gynaecological conditions 'which are detrimental to them as mothers'.

Maternity and child welfare – the nation's priority?

The rhetoric about British motherhood was often not even put into practice. Less than forty MPs were present during most of the debate on the Maternity and Child Welfare Bill in 1918. The new law permitted local authorities to provide many services free – but none of this was compulsory; they were allocated a very tight budget from central government, which simultaneously sent out reminders about the embarrassingly high maternal death rate. In 1928, the *Labour Woman* newspaper estimated that only ninepence per head of the population was spent on maternity and child welfare, whilst £2 a head was spent on the army and navy.

● **What community health services are made available to women now?**

Clinic sessions are largely for pregnant women and under-fives. It is often a battle to find other services, such as cervical cancer screening. Women have been refused cervical smears on the grounds that they are under 35, or have had a smear within the last five years. Cost-benefit analyses are done to decide whether a screening programme is economically worthwhile. Meanwhile, over 2,000 women die of cervical cancer every year – deaths which might have been prevented by early treatment.

Clinics for pre-menstrual tension (PMT) and menopause are also rare. A PMT clinic at a London hospital was closed down – because it had so many patients that it couldn't cope!

Well Woman Clinics can help, but some concentrate entirely on tests for cervical cancer and breast cancer. What about varicose veins, migraine, asthma . . . ? Where can we get proper check-ups for *all* aspects of our health? (For the many campaigns now going on to set up Well Woman Clinics with broad interests, see Chapter 5.)

The 'revolt against motherhood'

If birth control and abortion had been easily available, women's health would have improved greatly. Why were governments, and many powerful people, so wary of providing these services?

Newman thought he could identify 'a growing disinclination for children' in 1929. A 1932 Government report on maternal mortality noted that women were getting 'less patient and uncomplaining, more intolerant of pain and discomfort'. The Ministry of Health sent a circular to health workers, telling them to calm women down, and 'emphasise the grave risks attending interference with the course of pregnancy'.

An Inter-Departmental Committee on Abortion was set up in 1938, and heard a huge amount of evidence about the suffering of women: one expert suggested that *at least* 90,000 illegal abortions were carried out each year. The logical conclusion would presumably have been to change the law. Instead, the Committee recommended that the law should be harsher: doctors should notify the police when a woman came to them with a septic abortion, and the woman should be prosecuted and made to reveal the name of her abortionist. Birth control advice should be severely cut back; women at clinics should be 'advised and encouraged . . . to have children as soon as their condition permitted'.

Was there a fear that, if women were allowed to choose when to have children, they would decide never to have them at all? As a judge had said in 1920, when giving a ten-year sentence to a professional abortionist: 'those who have as many enemies as the British Empire must for their own safety have plenty of children to meet those enemies in the gate.'

Others were scared about *over*-population, which often meant that they thought the working classes were breeding too fast, although they welcomed children of 'better stock'. Perhaps it was safer not to make contraception and abortion freely available, but to keep some official control over women's fertility?

Another concern may have been to limit women's sexual freedom. Marie Stopes's book, *Married Love*, was called a 'handbook of prostitution' – she actually suggested that married women could enjoy sex. Newman thought that contraception might be used for 'selfish debasement and the encouragement of undesirable habits'. Anti-birth control campaigners issued dire warnings, saying that contraception caused sterility and was an 'unnatural act' like murder.

● Is information about birth control and abortion being made available to women now?

It is only since 1967 that birth control clinics have had the power to help women for 'social' as well as 'medical' reasons, and to advise unmarried women.

Abortion remains a taboo subject. Today, the Government-funded Health Education Council still carries *no* leaflets on abortion.

• What do anti-abortionists say today?

Members of anti-abortion organisations such as SPUC and LIFE believe that abortion is murder. They constantly attempt to change the 1967 Abortion Act, which made abortion free and legal. SPUC and LIFE also visit schools and tell girls that abortion is murder. Is it right that they try to impose their personal beliefs on others in this way?

LIFE recently advertised in the *Nursing Times*: 'You have a citizen's duty to uphold the law. . . . Report cases of children being born alive in abortion operations. . . . Report to the Police, or to us.' This sounds similar to the harsh suggestions made in 1938, to prosecute women and health workers involved in abortions.

• Is 'population control' still a reality?

Sometimes black women are specially encouraged to use fertility control. One woman reported:

'My GP is more liberal in referring black women [for abortions] because he feels they "breed too much". He does not refer white women for abortions, nor does he prescribe the pill for them.'
(Abortion Tribunal Evidence, 1977)

Other black women have been sterilised or had a coil put in without their knowledge or consent.

The new contraceptive injection, Depo-Provera, banned in the USA, is being tested on women in poor areas of Glasgow, on Asian women in East London, and on millions of women in Third World countries. Often women are not told it is on trial. The side-effects are disturbing:

'In two years I went from size 34 to size 44.'

'I felt terrible – sick and dizzy. I never had a period. I went back to the hospital, I was so angry with them . . . then they said I needed tranquillisers!' (Co-ordinating Group on Depo-Provera, evidence to the hearing on Depo-Provera, April 1983)

Eugenics is very much with us today. Some authorities seem to think that disabled people should be eliminated from this society. In a national survey, consultants were questioned on what they thought to be the most important reason for abortions. Three-quarters of those questioned said 'an abnormal foetus'. One stated 'we're in a position now to be selective about which people we want in the world.'

Where did women go for medical help?

Women sought help from a variety of sources. Of those who answered the Women's Health Enquiry, 60 per cent paid to see a doctor when ill. Others went to the welfare centre, health visitor or district nurse, the chemist, or, officially, 'nobody at all' (neighbours or relatives perhaps?).

Many women found it easier to approach a health visitor or district nurse than a doctor. They might mention their own problems during a consultation about the children.

11   Weighing a baby: from the film *The Health of the Nation*, 1937
The Ministry of Health helped to make this film for general release to cinemas. This scene had the title '13 lb. 6 oz. – heavyweight champion!'
Was the woman being assessed in some way, as a 'mother for Britain'?

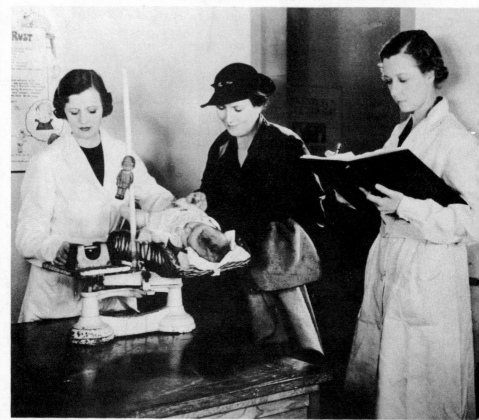

But women seem to have had contradictory feelings about health visitors. When a woman told the authorities that she was pregnant (notification was compulsory), the health visitor was supposed to make sure that there was no illegal abortion. As well as persuading women to accept motherhood, it was the visitor's official job to check how they treated their children. One sanitary inspector claimed that health visitors were there to help: after all, it was 'no reflection on a mother's love if Doris has managed to collect one or two nits in her hair'! However, notes were often sent from school, saying that children were dirty, or needed medical treatment which many women could not afford.

● Are women being monitored as mothers now?

In 1980, the Short Report (from a committee studying infant deaths) recommended that health authorities should establish what they called 'a commando group', including a health visitor and a community midwife, to encourage women to go to ante-natal clinics.

Health visitors can often give help and support to women. Yet part of their role is still supposed to be checking on women's behaviour. For example, some health visitors are issued with forms for 'Health Surveillance of Pre-School Children'. As well as ticking 'Yes' or 'No' for things like 'drinks from a cup', the visitor must simply tick 'Yes' or 'No' for 'Mother/Child Relationship Satisfactory'. A tick in the 'No' column could mean a close watch being kept over the woman in future.

Consultations with doctors

As for doctors, it seems that they did not give women much information. Although 750 women in the Women's Health Enquiry survey went to doctors for *treatment*, only sixty-seven of them said they obtained *advice* from a doctor. Marie Stopes was often told 'doctors are harsh and they do not know anything'.

Few doctors had ever experienced the living conditions of their working-class patients. At medical school they might have had one course of lectures in 'hygiene' and some discussion of sanitation and ventilation. The rest of their training was about curing people with 'interesting' diseases, rather than preventing basic health problems. A few radical doctors joined the Socialist Medical Association and the Campaign Against Malnutrition to protest about social conditions.

Most doctors showed little concern about the typical health problems of working-class women: anaemia, aching legs, headaches. Women reported comments like 'all women get back-ache around forty, so why worry', or (laughing at a woman in great pain from prolapse) 'tens of thousands of women are going about their work in a much worse state than you.'

Letters in Marie Stopes's book, *Mother England*, revealed that doctors acted particularly harshly towards women who asked about birth control:

> *'The doctor tells me it would be fatal if I became pregnant within two years, but gives no advice.'*

> *'When the last baby was born the doctor said "Can't you finish up" but when I asked him how he just laughed.'*

Other doctors (and nurses) seem to have given misleading advice about the rhythm method, and the use of douches and pessaries.

• Are doctors now more sympathetic to women's health problems?

Medical training is still geared towards illnesses which are seen as 'clinically interesting'. Many women find their symptoms are not taken seriously by doctors. A Well Woman Clinic worker commented: 'The number of women I've heard say, the doctor says it's just my age, this is just my problem. Some women come here absolutely desperate.'

Sometimes doctors hold moralistic attitudes towards women. The 1977 Abortion Rights Tribunal was told the story of a 16-year-old girl with an unwanted pregnancy:

> *'The consultant . . . refused to allow termination to take place until she was 18 weeks pregnant . . . he'd said to her "if silly girls like you are going to play around with sex you're going to pay for it". . . no pain-killing drugs were given to her until she had been in labour for about 18 hours.'*

Childbirth — beware the doctor

Medical attention at childbirth could be positively harmful to women. Doctors were often mentioned as being drunk and incompetent. One woman wrote: 'I have had the doctor's arm in my body, and felt his fingers tearing the afterbirth from my side.'

Although midwives were sometimes criticised too, doctors seem to have been especially dangerous. The high rate of death in childbirth amongst well-off women was often said to be because they got *more* medical attention! A book called *Mother Britain* drew on the notes of forty-five nurses and midwives: 'One needs eyes all round one's head adequately to supervise the doctor's movements,' even having to remind him to wash his hands to avoid passing on an infection. Midwives would avoid calling the doctor to home births if at all possible: 'you would practically tie a woman's legs together rather than get the doctor to sew her up,' said a Manchester midwife in the 1930s.

● Have advances in medical knowledge improved women's health?

Obviously some have done so. When sulphonamide drugs were introduced in the late 1930s, the maternal mortality rate dropped dramatically. Medical technology, used in the right ways, can be helpful to us, but we need to be aware of the problems it can cause as well. For example, during childbirth, women are often wired up to a machine which monitors the baby's heartbeat. The woman must stay lying down, even though it is known that labour would probably be shorter and easier if she could move around as she wished. Where these 'foetal monitoring' machines are used, medical staff tend to look at the machine instead of listening to the woman's own reports of what is happening, and doctors more often say a Caesarian is necessary.

The 'medicalisation' of ill-health

Bad medical treatment was not the basic cause of women's ill-health, although it certainly made things worse. However, medical facilities were sometimes made out to be the most important thing. Why was this?

A Government Committee on Maternal Mortality in 1932 compared women's health in Britain, Holland, Denmark and Sweden.

British women were the most likely to die in childbirth. They also had the worst general health; malnutrition, rickets (leading to a deformed pelvis) and infection in childbirth went together with poverty. However, the Committee ignored such evidence, saying that their task was to consider 'purely medical aspects'. As well as criticising women for not attending ante-natal clinics, they recommended more hospital facilities.

So, once again, attention was diverted away from living conditions. Even the British Medical Association and the Royal Commission on National Health Insurance said that money should be spent on fighting poverty rather than on more medical services. But to follow that advice could have ultimately meant major upheavals in society: it was more convenient to say that it was a lack of medical facilities – or women's failure to use them – which was at fault.

● **What suggestions are made to solve women's health problems now?**

Often, the 'magic answer' we are given is still a medical one. There are parallels between the 1932 Maternal Mortality Report and the Short Report of 1980, which looked at the reasons for infant deaths. Both examined how problems in pregnancy were connected with nutrition and living conditions. The Short Report admitted that 'in the long term, raising the standard of living is the best remedy'. The Committee then made 152 recommendations, all medical! The main ones were exactly the same as those of the 1932 report – encourage women to go to ante-natal clinics and intensify health education campaigns.

Quiz

This is a record of a discussion about women's experiences of the NHS. Again, the views are those of parents at a playgroup, women with small children, who answered the following questions:

1 Someone tells you that women live longer than men, so they must be healthier. Do *you* think

    (a) they're right

(b) women live longer because they're tougher

(c) women live longer because they don't do such dangerous jobs

(d) it's because of some other reason?

Everyone in the group answered (b)! There was a general feeling that men aren't necessarily more ill, they just complain more.

'The moment they've got a headache, they think they've got a brain tumour.'

'My husband, he got pains in his arm and chest one day and he wanted me to call an ambulance right away.'

'I think men, they're big babies when they're ill. I'd love them to have – not even a baby – just a period pain!'

It seems that men are very concerned about having heart attacks, for example, which may reflect the publicity about men needing to take care of their health. Women, on the contrary, are used to putting themselves last and never complaining.

2 Someone tells you that women are always complaining about their health – and it shows because women go to the doctor more than men. Do *you* think

(a) it's true that women complain a lot

(b) women have more time to go to the doctor for birth control, etc.

(c) women have to go to the doctor a lot with the children

(d) women get depressed more

(e) some other reason?

Nobody said (a). Most people said (b) *and* (c). One said (e).

Far from complaining, most women seemed reluctant to go to the doctor.

'Don't like going to the doctor. I never go for myself.'

'I get all wound up.'

'I go so often for my kids that I feel embarrassed going again for myself.'

Many avoided going because they found that the doctor often didn't take their illnesses – or their children's – seriously:

'I think they make you feel you're neurotic taking the children anyway half the time. When you call the doctor out you ask yourself, are they ill enough to have brought him out.'

'I phoned up twice in one week because my little boy was having croup – I was terrified. He shouted at me – he said: It costs me £4 every time someone calls me out.'

3 In the last six months have you gone to

(a) the baby clinic

(b) the dentist for your children

(c) the dentist for yourself

(d) a check-up for yourself (smear test, breast exam, etc.)?

There was a mixture of answers. One woman had had to beg for a cervical smear test, and if she hadn't made a scene and insisted, she wouldn't have got one.

Being examined or treated at a clinic had sometimes been off-putting:

'When the doctor put the speculum in it hurt and I told her, and she said well that shows it's in properly.'

Everyone thought there should be more Well Woman Clinics:

'definitely, many more.'

'the only one round here is at . . . and I only know about it because I work there, it's very busy anyway.'

4 It's a bad day, the kids are screaming and you haven't had time to tidy up. Your health visitor knocks at the door. Do you

(a) feel thankful she's come, because you need some help

(b) feel embarrassed

(c) ask her in

(d) ask her to come back another time?

Most people said (c). One person said (b) and two said (d). Nobody answered (a).

'You'd ask her in, but hope she'd see you were in a state and go' (this remark caused some laughter!)

Health visitors were thought to be 'a good idea for reassurance'.

'I know some people who go to the clinic every week with their first baby.'

'I did – I felt I needed someone to talk to.'

However, people felt that some health visitors didn't have a very helpful attitude:

'They go completely by the book.'

'They try to tell you you're doing it all wrong and they've not had one themselves.'

5 You go to the baby clinic and the health visitor says your baby hasn't put on much weight. Do you

(a) not worry – all babies are different

(b) worry that you're not feeding her properly

(c) ask the health visitor for some advice

(d) feel like not going back to the clinic again?

Most people said (a). One person said (b) as well – which maybe shows that even though women know babies are different, it's hard not to feel that you *might* be doing something wrong. One other person said (b), one said (c) and one said (d).

In discussion, more people admitted they would worry:

'You feel so guilty.'

'After they've told you your baby's underweight you remember it every time you feed her.'

'I was told he hadn't gained anything in two weeks, I worried myself sick, when I went back two days later she said, oh the scales were wrong that day.'

'Yes I've heard this a lot, that the scales are wrong.'

Several women also felt that child development tests were applied rigidly and often wrongly; again, they were made to feel nervous unnecessarily:

'They tend to compare, they used to compare my two. David hardly ever said a word and he was backward in their eyes, but he walked at ten months and he did things Jane couldn't do, so I said look two children are never alike. At one time I was even going to take David to the hospital, I was worried he was backward.'

'When they gave mine the hearing test he just wasn't listening, so they said he might be deaf – he's got to go through a whole course and finish that course before they can write it down that he's OK – well I know he's OK but I let them get on with it.'

6 You're pregnant and you see a poster telling you to go to the ante-natal clinic so that you'll have a healthy baby. Do you think

    (a) they're right, I'd better go so my baby will be healthy

    (b) I don't think going to the clinic makes that much difference to whether my baby's healthy or not

    (c) I don't feel much like going

    (d) that poster's a waste of time, I know that anyway?

Most people said (a). One said (b) and one said (d).

'I don't think the clinic's the main thing, not really.'

'They're good at detecting things, like blood sugar problems.'

'Oh yes, for all that side of it.'

'. . . but other than that, keeping yourself healthy, it's just being sensible.'

Although people thought they *should* go to the clinic, they didn't have all that much faith in medical experts, having had so many bad experiences:

'They said you've got a very small baby and lots of fluid . . . when David was born he was 10 lb. 14.'

Several women had had the same experience:

'They told me your baby's very small, I was worried sick, and she was ten pounds!'

'They say that they know when they don't know.'

Some medical workers were seen to be separating themselves off from women's experience:

'My baby was going to be breech so I said I want you to turn it and they said it's too late, so I rang my GP and he turned it perfectly easily and I had a normal delivery. Later the midwife came to me and she said, I understand how you feel now, I've just found out mine is feet down and I can't bear the thought of a breech delivery.'

'This is what I think, with some of them, they don't realise what you're going through.'

Several women had suffered from the strict application of the consultant's favourite regime for breastfeeding and baby-care:

'My breasts were so sore but girls in the other ward were given sprays. I asked the sister for one and she said what ward are you on, and I said Dr . . . .'s, and she said oh no, it's more than my job's worth, you don't need them. . . . he didn't believe in pain-killers or anything like that.'

Two women had been amused by a famous pro-breastfeeding paediatrician:

'so when Dr . . . . looked at her he said "Well, I'd say she was a breastfed baby" and I said – well she wasn't!'

'Well my baby had a terrible rash and he [same doctor] pulled her nappy off and he'd got all the students round him, I've never seen anything so funny, and he said "this is obviously a cow's milk rash" so I said thanks very much, I'm breastfeeding!'

'Everyone on the ward was petrified of him.'

'He's like a god to most people.'

'They're so pro-breastfeeding: women should have the option.'

7 You go to the doctor with a bad headache. He says you're depressed and wants to put you on tranquillisers. Do you

(a) take the pills

(b) tell him you want something else to stop the pain

(c) ask him for advice about any problems you may have (bad housing, no help with the kids, etc.)?

Half the group said (a) and half (c). One person ticked (a) *and* (c). One said (b).

'They tend to tell you everything's depression.'

'I went with a pain, he examined me and said there was nothing the matter, he said you've got an anxiety problem. . . . I didn't think so.'

Maybe some doctors are diagnosing depression too often now, and ignoring some physical illnesses?

Can doctors help you over the problems in your life?

'I don't think they can solve your problems but they can make you feel better if they talk to you about it.'

'My doctor wrote a letter about my housing – it did help.'

'My sister-in-law asked for a letter and the doctor said if you want a letter you can try the Medical Council, that was his attitude. She walked out of there really depressed.'

'Once my doctor said to me, just go home and go to bed, and I said how can I, I've got two children.'

'My friend, she looks really rough, with three small kids, she doesn't need someone to sit and talk to her and say "you should do this" . . . she needs physical help, she needs someone to actually give her a hand.'

As can be seen, most women had been through some difficult encounters with the health service, although they had good things to say about it as well. Everyone seemed to find relief in talking about their experiences. On many occasions, women had bravely stood up for themselves and insisted on what they wanted, despite the odds. Some more experiences are quoted in Chapter 5, 'How things might be changed'.

Suggested action

1 Ask older women what health care was like before the NHS. How often did they visit a doctor?

2 When you're going to the doctor, write down the questions you want to ask (your women's group could make suggestions). Make sure everything the doctor says is clear. If something is prescribed make sure the doctor explains what it is. If you don't want drugs ask for other forms of treatment. Can the doctor refer you for homeopathic treatment, for example? Take a friend with you when you see the doctor if this gives you more confidence.

3 Act out common situations in a group – one person can be the patient and another the doctor. The rest of the group looks on and gives advice. Some suggestions: asking for an IUD (coil) to be taken out, requesting an abortion, asking for a housing letter. In the acting you could try saying the things you'd *really* like to say, but find difficult in the real situation.

4 Watch out for private hospitals being built in your local area. Support campaigns to keep NHS hospitals and clinics open – otherwise we'll soon be paying for all our health care!

5 Arrange a group visit to your local Family Planning Clinic, or Brook Advisory Clinic for young people. Ask to discuss contraceptive methods with a worker there. You could probably do the same with other health facilities: for example, a social health worker could explain what happens at a Special Clinic (which gives help with problems like thrush, cystitis, and sexually transmitted infections).

6 Visit your Community Health Council's office – ask what it is doing about women's health issues. Can your group have a representative on the CHC?

7 Campaign for facilities for cervical smear tests (there are some mobile caravans, for example) to visit your area or your workplace.

8 Ask older women about their experiences of childbirth. What

were home deliveries like? Find out about the new drugs and machinery used at hospital births now. What are the advantages and disadvantages, based on the experiences of women you know?

9 Make up a questionnaire about what local women would like in a Well Woman Clinic (for women's general health). Take the answers to your Community Health Council (clinics have been set up in some areas as a result of women's campaigns).

A WOMAN'S JOB

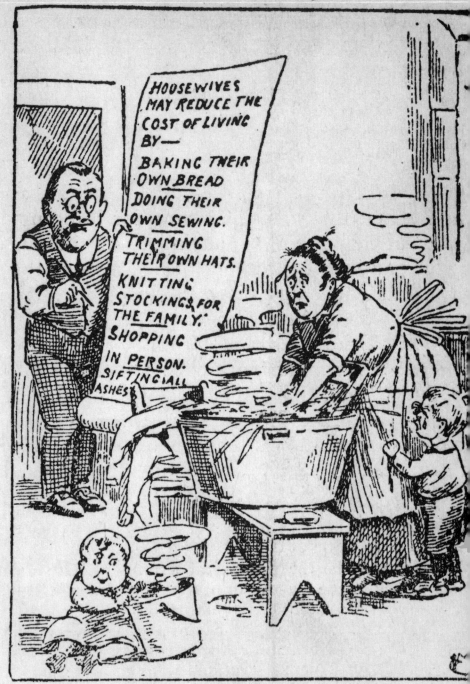

Tired Housewife: "Oh! thanks."

Chapter 3

DOES THE GOVERNMENT LOOK AFTER OUR HEALTH?

Introduction: Women are a cheap support system

People's welfare is either looked after by women – or by the State. If the State does not provide, it is assumed that women will do so. The authorities know that we will work extra hard to manage in bad housing, to feed the family on Supplementary Benefit, to look after elderly parents and disabled children who have nowhere else to go. Women are the end of the line.

Yet when a Government* makes policies about housing or Social Security benefits, they rarely mention all the work done by women at home. As for the effect of such a heavy responsibility on our health – that is never discussed. Women are officially 'forgotten'. Perhaps they cannot afford to remember us – it is cheaper to rely on women's work than to provide decent welfare services.

And if full welfare services came to be seen as a right, maybe women might start to feel less responsible. It is safer for the State to be able to call on our sense of duty whenever necessary.

Should women continue to accept this situation? Isn't it time that Governments worked to create a healthy society with full consideration of our needs?

Women as second-class workers

Officially, women were not seen as workers who deserved to be paid. At home, they worked in unhealthy conditions for nothing. And, in

(* It is important to say that Labour Governments, historically and more recently, have had a greater commitment to providing good living conditions than have Tory Governments. However, welfare policies promised in election manifestos have not always been carried out. Also, Labour Governments have sometimes cut back on services (although not as much as Tory Governments have done) which means they have constantly relied on women to cope.)

12 'A Woman's Job': from *Woman's Dreadnought*, 13 January 1917
The newspaper (which was produced for women in East London) obviously did not think much of this kind of advice. Do officials expect women to 'manage' in a time of difficulty?

other jobs, they worked in equally unhealthy conditions for next-to-nothing, because they were said to be casual workers, whose real duty lay in making homes for their families.

A Government report on South Wales in 1934 stated:

> '*Unemployment amongst women in South Wales does not present a very serious problem, so far as numbers registered at Employment Exchanges may be taken as reflecting the position. Apart from a comparatively small number of openings in the tin-plate trade, no industrial openings for women have ever existed in the area.*'

So women could not lose jobs because they had never had any in the first place! As for the Employment Exchange statistics, no wonder they showed so few women. It was difficult for married women to register as unemployed, because they had to satisfy strict rules to prove that they were 'genuinely seeking work'. Women could be said to be financially dependent on other people in the household. Often they had to do domestic work for low pay to prove they needed a job.

Such Government regulations supported a system in which employers could treat women badly. Most women left their jobs or were sacked when they got married. They were absorbed into a pool of unemployed people, and employers drew them out whenever it was convenient to do so.

For example, in the 1930s women were the source of profits for companies running new industries. Engineering, chemical manufacture, and canning were said to be especially suitable jobs for women. Employers claimed that women worked quickly, with nimble fingers, and were more obedient than men. They could also be paid much less. In 1931, women in engineering had average earnings of 27s.6d. a week. Men earned 52s.6d.

Employers and the Government made sure that women had little self-confidence, and saw any job, however unhealthy and low-paid, as a favour:

> '*A girl gave over at our mill last week; she told the manager she was not going to work for nothing. The manager said there were lots he knew would do the same if they thought they could sign on, showing that he knew how things are.*' (woman weaver from Lancashire)

● Is women's work valued equally with men's today?

The Labour Government introduced the Equal Pay Act in 1970. Yet employers have been able to get around this, because they only have to pay equally where women do the same work as a man, or work broadly similar to that of a man; employers can simply say women and men are doing different work. In fact, women work mainly in service industries, doing jobs very like their work in the home – cleaning, cooking, looking after the boss.

The European Court of Justice has ruled that the UK Government must change the Act because it should be possible to claim equal pay for work of equal *value*. However, will a tribunal be likely to consider that the kind of jobs women usually do are as valuable as those done by men?

In 1977, women's average pay was 75 per cent of men's. By 1979, the gap had *increased*.

● **Are women still seen as having less right to unemployment benefit?**

A Tory Government wants to emphasise the idea that women have little right to paid work. Patrick Jenkin, as Secretary of State for Social Services, said 'If the Good Lord had intended us all having equal rights to go out to work and to behave equally, you know he really wouldn't have created man and woman.'

Women are now 40 per cent of the labour force. Many women work part-time. Yet unemployment benefit officers have the discretion to refuse the dole to a woman if they decide that she is jeopardising her chances of employment, for example by only being available for part-time work, or by not having childcare arrangements which the officer considers satisfactory. Meanwhile, Government nurseries are being cut back.

Cutting benefit

In the first big depression, in 1921, there were 1.8 million registered unemployed. In 1931 there were 2.8 million. Governments made every attempt to pay out as little benefit as possible.

Through the infamous Means Test, a person's unemployment benefit was reduced if anyone else in the household was working. Furniture in the house might be valued and benefit reduced accordingly. When word spread that the Means Test officers were on their way, women quickly moved their furniture into neighbours' houses to try to escape this harsh rule.

If any doubt could be thrown on someone's eligibility for benefit, they had to appear before a Public Assistance Committee. Often benefit was cut or refused. A hunger marcher in 1936 told of women being asked whether they were breastfeeding – if they answered yes, they were given less money for their children's food.

In order to qualify for benefit, people were often forced to take jobs on Government projects; the Government got the use of cheap labour to clear land, do heavy building work – and even make furniture for Poor Law offices! Men were sometimes sent away to labour camps, known as 'slave camps', leaving women with the equally exhausting task of coping at home.

● **How are unemployed people treated by the State today?**

In 1982, with the number of unemployed at over 3 million, the Tory Government started to tax unemployment benefit. Meanwhile, by April 1983, 7 million people (the highest number ever) were

13   Unemployed women march to a demonstration in Hyde Park, 1920 The placards spelt out clearly that these women thought they had a right to paid work, or to a decent level of unemployment benefit. Why did they have to make such a protest – especially after the jobs they had done during the war?

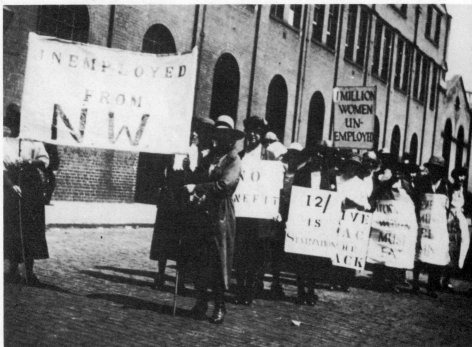

dependent on the welfare state's last resort, Supplementary Benefit – the official poverty line.

In a 1980 House of Commons debate on Social Security, Margaret Thatcher had said: 'I believe that it is right to have a larger difference between those in work and those out of work.' Of course, this difference makes people desperate to take even the worst jobs on offer. Unemployed people are pressurised to take jobs on schemes such as those organised by the Manpower Services Commission, through which the Government and private firms get work done for very low wages. These jobs often have a bad safety record too.

In fact, Governments have shown little commitment to making sure that healthy jobs are provided in Britain in general. There have never been enough factory inspectors (some work-places are only inspected once every seven years). When firms *are* brought to court for making employees work in dangerous con-ditions, the fines are usually tiny. 'Crown property' (which includes hospitals) is exempt from prosecution anyway.

The 'science' of nutrition

In 1933, the Minister of Health was told to decide how many calories a day a worker needed to survive. This was to be the basis for calculating how much unemployment benefit people should get.

Since the Government wished to set benefit as low as possible, it was obviously convenient if the number of calories needed was 'proved' to be very low. There was distinct embarrassment when the Ministry of Health said the adequate diet was 3,000 calories per man per day, whilst the British Medical Association estimated 3,400 calories.

An official conference was held to heal the breach. The two sides managed to emerge as a united front. They claimed to have discovered that the BMA's recommendations were for unemployed people, who were burning up calories as they tramped around seeking work. In fact, the original BMA report had said the opposite: that unemployed people were *less* active, and 3,400 calories was the rate for not very strenuous work! 'Scientific facts' seem to have been invented to suit the authorities.

The conference finally stated that a man doing heavy work needed 3,400–4,000 calories a day, an 'active' woman needed 2,800–3,000 calories, and a 'housewife' only 2,600–2,800! The experts considered housework a leisurely activity – although the original BMA report had

had the grace to admit that 'it cannot be assumed that the working man's wife leads a sedentary existence during the time her husband is out of work'.

Most unemployed people were receiving less money than they would have needed to buy even this minimum diet. This was a further source of embarrassment to the Ministry of Health. However, they referred to their 'scientific' guidelines in a general way, backing up policies which were causing widespread hunger.

• Is benefit enough now to provide a healthy diet?

William Beveridge, who planned the Social Security system which began after the Second World War, estimated how much food people needed by referring to the subsistence diets recommended in the 1930s. He based his calculations on 1938 prices. Between 1938 and 1948 the cost of living rose by 73 per cent. But benefits were only updated by 56 per cent. Since then, Supplementary Benefit has been increased periodically – but not in line with earnings.

The DHSS has made no further attempt recently to assess what would be a reasonable standard of diet. So are today's claimants expected to follow diets laid down in the 1930s – or, by now, to manage on even less?

A lack of healthy food

When women in working-class areas went shopping, they could usually only find expensive, poor-quality food. Firms distributed their goods to areas where they expected to make money. So brown bread, fresh meat, milk, fish and vegetables were hard to get in poorer areas. The Government did not intervene in the distribution system until the Second World War, when there was a sudden concern for working-class people's health. When ration books came in, many people's diet *improved*, because they received better food than before.

The Campaign Against Malnutrition pointed out that Ministry of Health reports encouraged people to buy good-quality food; however, the Ministry had not introduced laws to force the milk market to produce pure milk, or to stop the makers of tinned peas from putting harmful dye in their products. The companies continued to make profits from unhealthy food.

Food shortages were often artificially created. British farmers received State subsidies: they then produced less and kept prices high. Meanwhile, when ships reached British ports, they preferred to dump food in the ocean rather than to pay the high import tariffs. And in 1935, the Potato Marketing Board, a Government concern, 'experimented' with clearing its stocks cheaply to the unemployed – in order to decide whether this was financially worthwhile, or whether the potatoes should simply be destroyed.

John Boyd Orr, a well-known researcher on diet, said that poor nutrition due to poverty was a major cause of ill-health: the Government took no interest in his work.

• Is good quality food available to us now?

A lot of the food we buy is more harmful than we realise.

Eating sugar causes people to be overweight, and thus more likely to suffer from heart disease, high blood pressure, and diabetes. It also causes tooth decay. We eat, on average, almost 2 pounds of sugar a week each! Many foods contain 'hidden sugar' – for example, tinned soups and baked beans. The food industry encourages us to have a sweet tooth – to buy chocolate and fizzy drinks which make us crave even more sugar.

Food companies also add chemicals to their products; it is cheaper to preserve meat with sodium nitrite than to use refrigeration – but sodium nitrite has been banned in the USA because it is thought to form substances which can cause cancer. And tartrazine, which is used to colour orange squash, can trigger off allergic reactions.

As for foods which lack fibre (roughage), one good example is white bread. Firms make profits from white flour because they can sell the bran and wheatgerm separately (often as animal food). Meanwhile, diseases ranging from piles and constipation to tumours of the bowel seem to be caused by not eating enough fibre.

• Is the Government concerned to provide healthy food?

The Ministry of Agriculture is responsible for food safety. But its committees include representatives from the food industry. To make decisions about additives, the Government consults scientists who are also employed by food companies.

In the EEC, farmers pressurise Governments to pay them

high prices for milk, butter, and beef. The high prices encourage farmers to produce more and the result is 'lakes' of milk and 'mountains' of butter – but prices in shops don't necessarily fall. The EEC has even planned incentives to get people to eat more sugar! So food production is still not organised according to people's needs.

Government bodies rarely admit that our health is being harmed by food. In summer 1983, the *Sunday Times* revealed that the James Report, on goals for good nutrition in Britain, had not been officially released – due to pressure from the food industry. (The original report had suggested that our national diet should cut down on sugar – by half – and on fats and salt, and increase in fibre.)

Meanwhile, in institutions such as hospitals and schools, wholemeal bread and fresh fruit are not often found on the menu.

Housing – in short supply

After the First World War, the Ministry of Reconstruction was set up to build a new Britain: 'Homes Fit For Heroes'. There was a severe housing shortage – officially estimated at half a million houses.

The Ministry urged local authorities to start a building programme, which soon became chaos. For example, there were still 26,000 applications for 4,000 council houses in Birmingham in 1923.

Why was this? Often the Government backed out on its promises of money for local areas. Or money was given to private builders, who directed it towards housing for richer people. Only one-third of houses built privately with Government subsidies under the 1919 Housing Act were tenanted by working-class people.

In 1932 the Government stopped subsidising local authorities altogether, supposedly to stimulate private enterprise: but private companies still had no desire to build for working-class tenants, especially in the poverty-stricken Distressed Areas, where new housing was needed most.

Labour MP Ellen Wilkinson described a typical situation in Jarrow. As part of a slum clearance scheme, new housing had been built, but owners of the property prevented the Council from allowing the houses to be occupied. Women from the slums used to push their prams up the road to look in on the empty houses and imagine what it would be like to live there.

• Is the Government spending enough money on housing now?

Britain's housing problems are currently growing worse. In 1974/5 the Labour Government spent 96p on housing for every £1 on defence. By 1983/4 the Tory Government planned to be spending 33p on housing for every £1 on arms.

A 1980 House of Commons Committee warned that, at current rates of building, Britain would be short of half a million homes by 1985. Meanwhile, Environmental Health Officers reported that, in 1980, slum clearance work dropped, and the number of houses unfit for human habitation in England and Wales *increased* by 121,586. 'These places hadn't been wired for 38 years – it was unsafe. We had to fight for it to be done after there were four fires because of it.' (woman tenant from Liverpool)

The design of housing

The Ministry of Reconstruction approved plans for housing which was cramped, with few facilities. In 1920, the excellent new housing scheme of Newbury Borough Council was said by the Ministry of Health to be *too* good! Even in 1936, on the model new Grosvenor Estate built by the City of Westminster, the bath was put in the kitchen.

Suburban housing estates were officially praised for their healthy surroundings. Yet the houses were often badly built, and essential services like shops and community centres were sometimes not provided at all. It was expensive to travel to town to work or go shopping; so women were left with even less money, and a hard and lonely struggle to survive.

• Is housing better designed now?

Today one of the biggest housing problems is dampness. A recent survey by the National Consumer Council found 6 million damp houses in Britain. Where there is damp, it is usually women who battle against it, cleaning mould off the walls over and over again.

Another problem is tower blocks, which have proved the worst kind of environment for most people – depressing, inconvenient and dangerous.

Dampness and high-rise flats often go together. They are typical of Council housing built in the 1960s, when the Labour

Government was desperate to create as many homes as possible, as cheaply as possible. They turned to private contractors, who were eager to make profits by building shoddy, concrete-block housing without proper insulation.

In April 1982, Sedgefield District Council in County Durham decided to demolish a block of flats built in 1969. Known locally as 'Colditz', the flats had suffered from damp ever since being built. It was cheaper to start again (at a cost of £4 million) than to do repairs. The Council accepted £120,000 from the contractors who built the flats, instead of taking them through the courts.

Some housing estates have won design awards, but turned out to be impossible to live in because of damp – such as the Mozart Estate in Westminster. And many new towns, advertised every-where as a desirable place to live, are still without essential services.

● What is officially said about the effect of housing on our health?

Almost nothing! Since 1974 the health services and the housing services have been separate. The Ministry of Health between the wars did at least deal with housing *and* health services – the connection between them was officially recognised.

Even if you can get an expert to say that housing is damaging your health, it is very difficult to get re-housed. There is always a long list of council tenants waiting for a transfer for medical reasons: 'Our doctor wouldn't give my kid a chest X-ray in case it was positive. He said he'd have hundreds of people asking for them then.' (woman from Liverpool)

Helping women out?

Why were women so rarely given help by the State with their task of running the home?

Municipal wash-houses were very popular, but there were not nearly enough – in Liverpool, six places were used by a third of a million women, who often had to wait for hours. When Fulham Council set up the Fulham Mechanical Wash in 1920, women were overjoyed because they could leave their washing in a bag and collect it later. But the Council was taken to court by Fulham laundry-owners – and the Justice ruled that it was against the law for the Council to wash

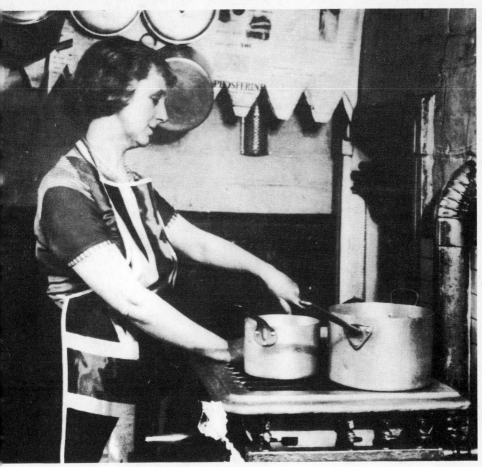

14 Mrs Constance Whitham in her kitchen, Manchester, 1937, wearing a
silk apron commemorating the Silver Jubilee
Women have always worked hard at home – often with little recognition –
and the country has benefited from this work.

clothes for women, although it was legal for them to provide facilities
for women to do the work themselves.

Mine-owners refused for years to provide pit-head baths – they
wanted miners to save them money by washing at home. But women
pressed constantly for these facilities, since they felt that, as one woman
said, 'the miner's wife in present conditions is little better than a slave.'

Home-help services were seldom provided by Councils, who
often made the excuse that 'women did not want them'. In fact,
well-organised services, like that of Edmonton Council in 1935, were

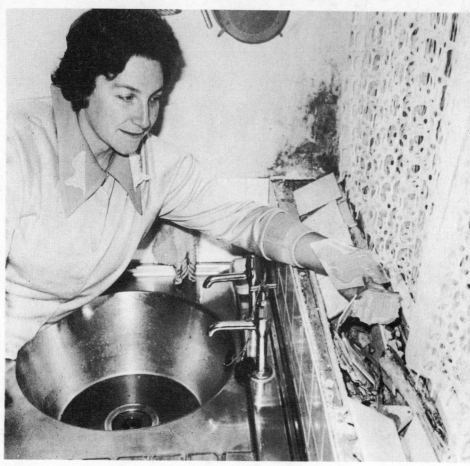

15 'Mrs. Wayne's windowledge – typical of many houses on her estate',
Labour Weekly, 24 June 1977
Why have women, on top of everything else, had to deal with bad living
conditions such as the damp kitchen shown here?

accepted with satisfaction by women – although it did take time for
them to get used to the idea.

National Kitchens were provided in the First World War – British
Restaurants and nurseries were provided in the Second World War, so it
obviously was possible for the Government to arrange communal
facilities which would cut down tremendously on housework. It was an
efficient way to run a society, and enable women to do other jobs. But
in peace-time women were expected to take over again at home.

Was this because it was cheaper for the authorities if women did the
work themselves? Or was it also because, in this way, women would

continue to concentrate their energies on their homes and families, with little expectation of any change?

- ## Who cares for people now – women? or the State?

Even though we have a much wider Social Security system than in the 1930s, that system was never designed to take full care of people in need. William Beveridge, who planned the scheme, wrote in 1942: 'the great majority of married women must be regarded as occupied on work which is vital though unpaid . . . without which the nation could not continue.' This was one of the rare occasions on which women's contribution was officially mentioned, and it was only a mention. It was also a statement of an intention to leave women alone to cope. 'National Kitchens' have not been seen since the Second World War. Home-help services and public wash-house facilities are being cut back or closed down.

Many women look after sick and disabled relatives at home, with little or no financial help. When the Equal Opportunities Commission began a survey of 'carers' in 1980, they advertised in women's magazines. Ten thousand women wrote in. The EOC noted that: 'A striking factor was the repeated expressions of simple gratitude from correspondents who had felt themselves to be worthless and forgotten.'

The ultimate insult comes to married women who are looking after a disabled relative. They have no right to receive the Invalid Care Allowance because you can claim this only if you have 'given up work' to do the caring, and it is *assumed* that married women don't work in the first place!

As the Government cuts back on day centres, nurseries, and hospitals, women face yet more burdens. A woman with a disabled child wrote to the EOC:

> *Of course I could put my daughter into hospital and lead a normal life. This would cost the Government a lot more. . . .*
> *The Government, whichever party is in power, have a great pool of cheap second class labour, the mothers and housewives.'*

- ## Why are women sometimes glorified as 'heroines'?

On 7 February 1979, the *Daily Mirror* carried a front-page headline, 'The Unsung Heroines'. A woman, said the *Mirror*, 'is the mainstay of her family and the backbone of the nation. When her husband goes to work she has nothing to do all day . . . except cook, shop, clean, dust, mend, tend . . . and fetch and carry.' At last, a recognition of women's hard work? Perhaps – but there was no suggestion that other people should share that work. The *Daily Mirror* clearly thought women should carry on doing all this – it was 'natural'. 'She is not as good as a man, but better. Not as strong, but stronger.' Maybe if women were praised to the skies for performing their traditional role, they might be stopped from complaining, insisting on help from others, or even joining Women's Lib!

The *Mirror*'s last word was a Heroines Competition; presumably men were to make the nominations – 'Do *you* know an unsung heroine? She could be a neighbour, a friend, your wife or your mother. Send your nomination, with a brief description of what makes her so wonderful, to. . . .'

We can only speculate as to what the prize was, but we know the prize in real life – physical and emotional exhaustion. Women pay dearly for the supposed 'reverence' for motherhood; we lose our health and our freedom.

Quiz

1 Do you think unemployment benefit and social security should be

(a) put up

(b) cut down

(c) stay the same?

Most of the group said (a). One said (c) and one wrote 'assess individually'. Everyone laughed at the idea of (b)!

Does unemployment cause extra stress for women?

'My husband was out of work for two weeks and the tension . . . not knowing what was going to happen.'

'My husband's only been unemployed two days and already he's in bed all morning . . . he's always leaving plates with crumbs around.'

'It irritates you so much if you're running around and they're laying there.'

2 Do you think the Government should spend

(a) less on defence and more on health, housing, education, etc.

(b) less on health and housing, and more on defence

(c) whatever their experts say?

Everyone said (a).

'They say trains go past here with nuclear waste twice a week – it's not properly inspected.'

'There should be more day nurseries and day centres – the money should go on that.'

'No Government's ever tried not spending any money on defence – it's remarkable, you'd think someone would give it a go for a few years or so.'

'But doesn't it keep a lot of people in employment?'

'But they could be building houses instead.' 'That's true.'

'Now we've got computers it's so easy to take national votes on big issues – we should be able to vote on individual policies – even if you vote a Government in, you don't know . . . obviously they change their policies.'

3 If you had more money would you

(a) spend more on food

(b) spend less time looking for bargains

(c) spend less time making and repairing clothes

(d) spend less time planning your weekly budget?

Most people said (d). Several said (a) and several (b). One person wrote 'Do less work'.

'Food's a priority then clothes.'

'You just have to have cheaper things to eat. I used to make stew with beefburgers.'

'My husband leaves it all to me, planning the budget. We both got really nervous when he was unemployed.'

'I've got family around – they help you through the hard times –

but I don't know what you'd do without them – I couldn't really ask friends.'

'Maybe in the past, people were more caring.'

'They enjoyed the neighbourly part of it sometimes – I think.'

Maybe women today feel more isolated with their burdens?

4 Your home is damp, and green mould has started to grow on your kitchen wall. Do you

- (a) find out if it's happening to your neighbours too
- (b) keep on cleaning the mould off
- (c) ask the Tenants' Association or Rights Centre what you can do
- (d) report it and wait for something to be done?

Most people said (d). A couple said (a) and a couple (c), and one said (b).

'I've got damp, the whole house has, it's private rented and the landlord doesn't want to know.'

'Our flats are brand new and they've got damp. A man came to fix it and he said, you're all right till it rains again – and I have to keep on cleaning the kitchen floor, it smells all musty.'

Several people thought housing was not designed safely enough:

'My friend, she was downstairs in someone else's flat doing the washing-up and suddenly she saw her little boy fall past the window – he lived but if that was me I'd crack up.'

'The sheltered housing they're building for old people now, they should build that for everybody.'

5 Wholemeal bread is better for health than white bread, but it's more expensive. Do you think the Government should

- (a) make wholemeal bread cheaper
- (b) keep white bread cheaper because people like it
- (c) not do anything about it (leave the prices up to the bread companies)?

Several people said (a) and several (c).

> *'My husband won't eat anything else. He's heard it's healthier.'*

> *'Mine won't eat it. I like it but I usually don't buy it because he doesn't like it.'*

> *'A white loaf looks more – but it doesn't fill you up much.'*

> *'The mills are set up to make white flour – it costs more to make brown bread.'*

> *'People should be able to choose, so long as you can get both of them and the prices aren't too different.'*

6 The Council's going to close the nursery where your child goes. Would you

(a) accept that your child's going to be at home with you now

(b) think 'I suppose they have to save money somehow'

(c) join together with other parents to complain

(d) try and get another nursery opened somehow?

Everyone said (c) or (d).

> *'I think we'd be all right round here, we'd manage because we'd get together and do something – like the playgroup.'*

> *'You do need nurseries and playgroups though, it's a real strain if the kids are with you all the time.'*

7 Women don't get paid for looking after their children or their elderly parents. Do you think

(a) it's women's duty to do that anyway

(b) it's a valuable job and women should be paid for it

(c) men should help more

(d) there should be more nurseries and day centres?

Most people said (d). A couple also said (b) and (c). One person wrote 'family should work together'.

> *'I don't think you should be paid for looking after your children – it's your choice to have them.'*

'I never thought about being paid – it would be nice though.'

'It's a 24-hour job.' 'It's true you're always working.'

'With elderly people, especially if they're ill, I think it's different. Maybe you should be paid for that.'

'You really need all the day centres and things.'

'My husband's the helpful kind so it does make a difference.'

'It's not very helpful is it, just to say women are wonderful. We need more help really.'

Suggested action

1 Ask older women what it was like living through the 1930s and 1940s. What changes happened for women during the Second World War – more jobs? more nurseries? Did those changes last after the war ended?

2 Find out about your rights to welfare benefits. Contact a Citizens Advice Bureau or local Law Centre. Make sure you are getting *everything* you're entitled to.

3 Write a questionnaire about housing problems and take it round the area where you live. What are the common difficulties and what is their cause – wrongly designed housing? no repairs being done? repairs done badly? Can an Action Group or tenants' group, in association with a local Law Centre, use the results of the questionnaire to publicise the problem and press for something to be done about it?

4 Join a union at your workplace, if possible, and ask for training on the TUC health and safety courses. Help to check your workplace for hazards and, through your safety representatives, press for conditions to be improved.

5 Act out in a group situations such as: going to the Social Security Office to claim benefit, to the Housing Office to make a complaint, to a workplace safety committee to discuss a dangerous piece of machinery. The group can give encouragement and ideas to the people doing the acting.

6 Look at the labels on food (the ingredients are listed in order; the first one is the main one and so on). How many foods contain sugar? Which foods contain least sugar and least chemical additives? What is really in slimming foods and how much are you paying for them?

7 Visit your local bakers and ask if they sell wholemeal bread. If not, can a group of you as customers persuade them that it's a good idea? (Many bakers now *do* sell it because they realise that there's a demand for it.)

8 Cook together as a group – try out some new recipes, especially using wholefoods and vegetables (brown rice, brown pasta, beans, lentils, salads).

9 Ask older women – what did they do to make ends meet in times of difficulty? was there more community spirit in the past? did people rely more on family or friends? Have women become more isolated now? How can we help to support each other?

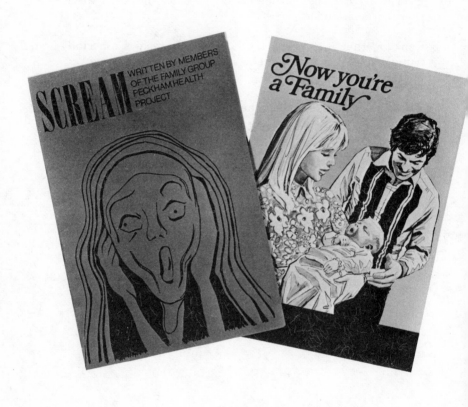

16 Different views of motherhood: cover pictures from a pamphlet written by a women's group, and from a health education booklet

Chapter 4

HEALTH EDUCATION
Laying the blame on women

Introduction: Health education can cause women harm

Education can be used to help us understand what is really happening in our lives, or to cover up the truth. Health education has often been used to make people think that illnesses are largely their own fault, for not having a healthy lifestyle. But in the last chapter we saw that society is not organised in a healthy way in the first place – people cannot 'choose' good housing or good food if none is provided.

At times of economic depression, when even more illness is being caused by poverty, bad housing, and malnutrition, a Government has a special interest in directing blame away from its own policies and towards other people. It's probably no coincidence that health education became very popular in the 1930s – and the Conservative Government is encouraging it now too.

Health education is directed mainly at women. After all, women are said to be responsible for keeping the family in working order. And it takes so little to make women feel guilty – many of us spend most of our lives worrying that we have not done enough. So health education sets up a competition for the best-kept house and family, for the perfect wife and mother. To succeed in this competition, you are told that you must have the advice of experts – the authorities do not want to recognise that women might actually be the experts on our own lives.

For all women, this kind of health education can cause worry and lack of confidence in ourselves. For women who are already battling desperately to cope in impossible conditions, it often comes as the final insult.

We certainly need more information about health – but of a very different kind. We need to understand how this society is dangerous to women's health. And each of us needs to decide what we can realistically do, under these difficult conditions, to increase our confidence and to work for improvements in our health.

Keeping an eye on women

Women often got advice about health from the local chemist, friends, or neighbours, said a Government report on maternal mortality in 1932. Janet Campbell, who wrote the report, was alarmed that women preferred to do this rather than go to a clinic – she thought they might be spreading 'old wives' tales' to each other. But although some popular ideas about illness might have been wrong, doctors *also* gave wrong information (for example, about birth control – see Chapter 2). In 1928, in a pamphlet called *The National Care of Motherhood*, the Women's Co-operative Guild had defended women's choice, saying that you could often get better advice on childbirth from neighbours than from male doctors, or from female doctors who hadn't had children.

People in authority obviously felt threatened by the idea that women might talk to each other and get health care outside the official health services. The Government and doctors were united against people using home remedies or getting medical supplies without visiting a doctor. The British Medical Association published books called *Secret Remedies*, in which they analysed what was in patent medicines, and said that most were a trick. Although this was probably true, the Association was also against many herbal remedies, which might have been very useful.

The authorities were especially worried about substances which women used to start abortion – like pennyroyal, a common herb. The Pharmacy and Poisons Act of 1933 put several such drugs on 'restricted sale'. This meant that a chemist could only sell them on prescription – or else get the person who bought them to sign the Poisons Book so that the Government had a record of the sale.

- **Are pressures put on women today to get all their health information from the experts?**

Most official health education material gives two clear messages: first, that medically trained people must always be your guide on health matters – and second, that women should avoid sharing problems with each other and exchanging advice.

The Health Education Council has issued a poster which asks 'How can another woman make you pregnant?' It goes on to say 'Just by talking to you. . . . Too many women risk getting bad advice about contraception because they'd rather listen to friends than go to a clinic or doctor.' The poster claims you can get advice that is 'friendly, private and above all accurate' from medical people. But, unfortunately, this is not always the case – and even when it is, why shouldn't women discuss contraception with each other *as well*?

● **What do the experts say when women get together to talk about health?**

In the past few years, women have begun to meet in groups to find out more about our bodies, talking about everything from diet, childbirth, and stress, to hazards at work, menopause, and depression.

Most of the women involved have no medical training. Some do, and want to share their knowledge openly. This Women's Health Movement has produced information which is vital. Books and leaflets have been written on common problems such as thrush and cystitis, giving simple remedies which have been found by the writers and their friends to be effective. This is the tradition of many of the so-called 'old wives' tales' – the way in which women exchange experiences to learn more about health.

Two women explained how a health course had helped one of them to cope with cystitis:

'I got a leaflet that says take a teaspoonful of bicarb of soda, and drink so many pints of water . . . tried it and it worked straight away.'

'She's had cystitis since she was 14 and now she's 22 – the doctor had put her on thousands of tablets . . . but after our women and health course she's hardly suffered since . . . and that was just talking.'

Many women have become interested in alternative forms of health care (such as homeopathy, acupuncture, osteopathy, naturopathy, herbalism). These use gentler remedies, and look at the person as a whole instead of as a machine-like body which can always be cured by technology.

Women's health groups have also provided a chance to compare experiences of medical treatment. A woman may discover, for example, that she is not the only one to have suffered pains or infections when using the coil for contraception – although her doctor might have told her to carry on and 'get used to it'. Health groups have been involved in campaigns against the dangers of contraceptives, like the Dalkon Shield (a type of coil). Women have also come to feel that many drugs are being wrongly used: Valium, for example, can be addictive, with alarming withdrawal symptoms – and is often useless in helping a person to cope with the real causes of depression.

Many medical experts respond by saying that it is 'dangerous' to do internal examinations for yourself and other women, or for 'untrained' women to fit caps. Yet women's groups learn carefully and slowly together – compare this to the fact that a doctor may have become qualified to give contraceptive advice with very little experience of fitting caps.

17   Pregnancy testing at Balham Family Centre
Many women's groups are now providing a free pregnancy testing service, in a friendly atmosphere. Women who come can see the result of their test immediately and talk about their feelings if they wish. Could health service clinics more often take this informal approach?

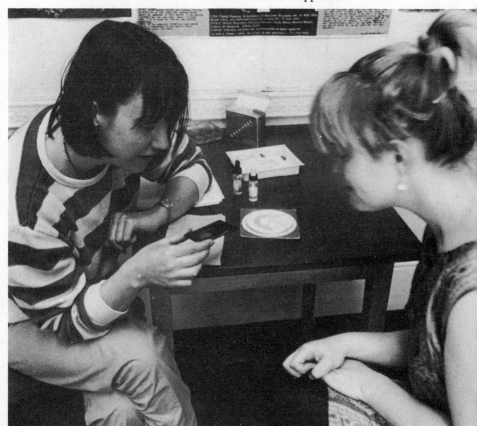

● **How are women treated who are used to doing their own health care?**

Knowledge about herbs and home remedies has largely vanished in this country. However, many women who have come to Britain from other countries have not yet lost their healing skills.

> *'When I was sick my grandmother used to go out and pick bush – herbs and plants, in the garden or growing wild. As I grew up I learned what to use too.'* (West Indian woman)

> *'For colic we gave lime-flower or orange peel – boiled.'*

> *'We used to give aniseed boiled in water – just give it plain. Oh yes, it worked well.'* (from a discussion amongst women of Third World origin)

Instead of learning from this store of wisdom, the British authorities instruct health education workers to tell black women 'how we do things here', from the standpoint that 'modern' ideas are superior:

> *'Some ethnic groups still cling to the old way of doing things, retaining their language, habits and culture ... sometimes help is required to develop new attitudes to health and the care of their family.'* (a doctor, in *Nursing Times*, 1978)

Often, women from other countries have helped at childbirth and learned some key things through experience: 'The usual way to give birth back home was squatting or sitting up. My mother had six of us that way. Never laid on her back.' (West Indian woman) After years of pressure from women's groups, this idea is only just beginning to be accepted in British hospitals.

Training the mothers

A special effort was made to convince women that, when it came to having children and bringing them up, expert advice was necessary. George Newman of the Ministry of Health talked of 'ante-natal supervision', meaning not only a medical check-up, but also a chance to persuade women to behave in certain ways. Janet Campbell wrote that during ante-natal care, each woman should gain 'a steady trust in those who are responsible for her safety and well-being' plus 'a healthy attitude of mind towards the future child'.

A Conservative Minister of Health, Hilton Young, said in 1934 that it was extremely important to make sure women received health education, since the need was for 'the right raw material' to 'grow enlightened mothers'. As a Manchester clinic said in a 'Notice to Mothers': 'The Infant Welfare Centre is not intended for the treatment of children who are ill, but is for the purpose of giving advice on the prevention of illness and the feeding and care of children.'

● **Is there a special focus on getting pregnant women to accept health education now?**

From the front page of *Baby* newspaper, produced by the Health Education Council, we learn that pregnant women need

> *'more advice than they'll get from just talking to their friends and family! . . . All through your pregnancy there will be a team of experts ready to help you. Your GP, midwife, hospital consultant and health visitor have "had" a lot of babies in their time.'*

The implication is that a male consultant knows more than a pregnant woman about every aspect of her situation.

The medical experts are also very concerned to tell women how to bring up children. Of all money spent directly on health education 80 per cent was spent educating mothers in childcare, wrote Susan Slovak (health visitor) in the *Nursing Times* in 1972. There is little change now.

● **Are men being enlisted on the side of the health professionals?**

The idea that men should be more involved in childbirth can be a good thing – but it may bring difficulties for women too. Some health professionals seem to want to make fathers the hidden persuaders: for example, about the benefits of technology. A recent American health education film on childbirth showed a woman who had strong feelings against the use of drugs arguing against the health staff *and* her husband, who were all trying to persuade her that, although the baby wasn't currently 'at risk', it *might* be soon if she didn't take the drugs.

A National Childbirth Trust leaflet tells future fathers to make sure their wives attend ante-natal classes – 'do encourage her to go' – and if a fathers' class is offered 'just go along to support your wife. You will learn many interesting facts so that you will be able to refute old wives' tales and horror stories . . . and so help to keep up your wife's confidence.'

This seems to encourage men to *undermine* women's confidence – to prevent us from believing in the reality of our own and other women's experiences. In contrast, women are rarely urged to rely on female friends or to have another woman present during childbirth.

Bombardment from all sides

To make sure that officially approved advice was handed out whenever possible, the Government gave its support to the army of health educators who might reach women outside the health services – in their homes, on the streets. George Newman urged all towns to follow the example of Plymouth, where, by 1927, there was a health magazine selling 10,000 copies a month, health advertisements on trams, and frequent lantern slide shows. Other towns had Health Weeks with exhibitions at the town hall, including commercial stalls. Companies such as Izal (selling disinfectant) were eager to join in and advertise their products.

Throughout the country, voluntary organisations like the People's League of Health and the National League for Health, Maternity and Child Welfare put up exhibitions and arranged health talks. In 1925, Newman listed twenty-three voluntary health societies in operation. Some were partly funded by the Ministry of Health.

Health magazines and health talks could have been useful – if they had been set up with a helpful attitude to women. But this was rarely the case.

• How is health education done today?

Officially information is supposed to be spread via Health Education Officers, employed by local Health Authorities. These officers are expected to contact health workers, teachers, community workers, and occupational health nurses in factories, for example, and arm them with materials produced by the Health Education Council, a central Government-funded body. Health exhibitions and advertisements are still a major activity, especially when there is a campaign about a particular issue (to stop pregnant women from smoking, to get people to take more exercise). Health education officers who criticise the content of national campaigns – for example, asking why large sums of money are being spent on promoting a bicycle race round Britain at a time of mass unemployment – have often had a cold reception from the Health Education Council.

Businesses are getting more involved in health education all the time. The Mars food firm, which makes sweets and chocolate, now has a Dental Health Education Department! Johnson and Johnson employs ex-health visitors to visit clinics and promote films such as 'Touch of Love', which explains how to massage your baby – using Johnson's Baby Lotion.

A patronising attitude to women

Most health education was done by people who did not live in the same circumstances as the women they wished to educate. They were part of a society which stereotyped working–class women as weak and feckless, a different breed from themselves. Eleanor Rathbone, women's rights campaigner, gave some typical examples of remarks made by the upper classes:

> *'Working women enjoy poor health.' 'They are used to it.'*

> *'They have no nerves and do not suffer like educated people.'*

> *'They like never being alone.'*

In Parliament, during a debate on whether shiftwork could harm women's health, Sir Frederick Banbury MP said that he didn't see why it should be a problem, because he had got up at six o'clock every day when he was at public school and never suffered from it!

Instead of congratulating women for the hard work they put into motherhood, health educators often expected women to accept a view of themselves as ignorant and lazy. Feminist Winifred Holtby noted the tendency in 'cheap journals and cheaper speeches' to suggest that modern mothers were neglectful. Rebecca West of the Labour Party was angry that the Ministry of Health should make the 'infamous assertion' that babies died because women were ignorant.

• How do today's health educators see their clients?

Many health education workers still look upon their clients as a race apart – the unconverted. Efforts are particularly directed towards working-class people, always called – usually in a patronising tone – 'Social Classes Four and Five'. A chief medical officer from Scotland said:

> *'This group is large and difficult to identify, and in terms of health education is the most difficult to influence. Interest of the individual is often transitory and motivation weak. Indeed, there is often a suspicion of any form of official advice at all. In many ways this group is the greatest challenge of all.'*

Recently, some health educators have started to talk about 'at risk groups' – which include poor people, black people, single parents and almost anyone else who is not white, middle-class, well-off and married. This can still be a way of singling out people who are seen as 'unfortunate', people who 'cannot cope' with this society – rather than looking at why society is unhealthy in the first place.

The impression is often given that people are unhealthy because they do not read health education leaflets, rather than because they live and work in bad conditions. This is a useful idea for a Conservative Government to promote. Patrick Jenkin, Secretary of State for Health, said to the British Medical Association in 1979, 'it is a perversion of good practice to allow, let alone encourage, people to live their lives in a way which seriously damages their health', but he was not attacking companies which build damp housing, nor was he about to announce that the Government would stop making money from taxes on cigarettes. Instead, he said: 'the cardinal principle must be to emphasise the individual's personal responsibility for his own health.'

• What is the attitude towards women in particular?

The tone of the health information for women is particularly patronising.

The *Pregnancy Care* card, in use until recently, has a space on the front for the pregnant woman (or even her doctor?) to write her name – surrounded by a frilly edge, looking like a nameplate in a children's book. The questions inside sound as though they are addressed to children too:

'Has my doctor confirmed that I'm pregnant?'

'Do I know when my baby's due?'

'Am I managing to keep my clinic appointments?'

Cartoons in *Baby* newspaper show women as laughing-stocks, with staring eyes and stupid expressions, either with sexy figures or looking dirty and run-down. Equally insulting is the poster of a woman with a dumb look on her face, with the caption 'Don't wait for your baby to prod you into going to the doctor!' – as if women are not intelligent enough to remember to go to the clinic.

Men are advised to see their wives as helpless creatures. A National Childbirth Trust leaflet for *Expectant Fathers* says: 'you come into your own when choosing major equipment such as a pram . . . it will be up to you to see that the brakes work and the handle is the right height for easy pushing.' It also suggests that the father's contribution to baby care should be 'to simplify the feeding, bathing and cleaning routines with the intelligent application of a little time and motion study'.

Housework is made out to be 'not real work' – it is something men can stoop to do occasionally: 'Even practical little things like helping with the domestic chores . . . can be invaluable to an expectant lady.' (*Baby* newspaper)

Irrelevant advice

The information which health educators tried to spread was often useless to women, given the conditions under which working-class people had to live.

To those living in slums in polluted cities, the People's League of Health offered lectures on *The Value of Sunlight and Pure Air*. The National Fitness Campaign, launched in the late 1930s, proclaimed the benefits of a healthy body – but the sports facilities which were supposed to come with the campaign were never provided.

The National League for Health, Maternity and Child Welfare leaflet, *To Expectant Mothers*, told women to have a hot bath daily (with a footnote saying 'in many homes this would be impossible, but it is included for those by whom it can be managed.') Another hint which working-class women would have found ironic was 'no heavy work should be done during the last month of pregnancy.'

Even more extraordinary were the Ten Health Commandments issued by the Women's Imperial Health Association some years earlier

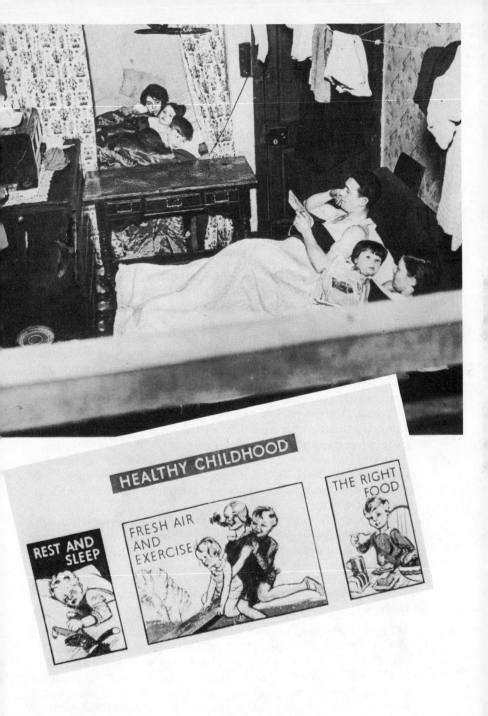

18a Family in Glasgow, c. 1938   18b   Health education posters of 1933
How could families living in such conditions achieve a healthy upbringing
for their children? How might women have felt on seeing these posters?

(in 1913). They included 'Drink good water, and eat plain wholesome food. Eat slowly, with plenty of time between meals. Choose a dry house. Cultivate temperance, early hours, and regular personal habits' and 'Always laugh when you can. Laughter is a cheap medicine.' Perhaps the only thing which would have given women a laugh was the shortsightedness of the Women's Imperial Health Association!

• Is health education advice more realistic now?

The main Health Education Council campaign recently has been 'Look After Yourself'. The message is that you can avoid illness if you take exercise and watch your diet.

The suggestions for exercise might be useful for business executives, but most women, looking after children and with little time or money, would probably find them ridiculous: 'don't dawdle on the golf course'? 'Take to the hills whenever you can'? 'Why stand in a bus queue – when with a bit of effort, you can walk almost as quickly'? Ironically, housework is even suggested as a keep-fit exercise: in a section called 'Choose *Your* Exercise', the *Looking After Yourself* booklet lists 'housework (moderate)' along with twenty-one types of sport!

As for the air you breathe when jogging, the Health Education Council takes no responsibility for this. A booklet called *How To Stay Alive* says that cigarette smoking is 'the most important source of pollution in Britain today'. The booklet aims to convince readers that ill-health is entirely their own fault; the moral is 'if you smoke, think twice before you complain about car exhausts and factory fumes!'

This fits in with recent attempts by the Government to play down the dangers of lead pollution. Perhaps the campaign should be called 'Look After Yourself – Because No One Else Will!'

• What advice is given about health problems common to women?

Many women have backache. The HEC leaflet *Mind Your Back* gives six reasons for back-strain. All of them point to 'bad habits' – bending down or lifting wrongly, being overweight. Nowhere does the leaflet consider the other causes of back-strain for women – carrying children up flights of stairs when the lift is out of order, working in hospitals where there are no mechanical hoists to lift patients. The leaflet finishes: 'if *you* do not take care of your *own* back you may be letting yourself in for years of pain . . . isn't it worth a little effort NOW?' Many women would say that their pain comes from having to make too *much* effort, not too little.

Another leaflet, on *Varicose Veins*, gives advice about treatment, but says nothing about prevention. The comment 'women are more often affected than men' is made, but this seems to be taken for granted (as a biological fact maybe, rather than as a result of all the time women are on their feet?).

Not working hard enough?

Nobody in authority wanted to take responsibility for providing healthy living conditions. The implication was always that if women failed to keep their families healthy, they were not working hard enough. Cleanliness, often more important to people's health than drugs and medical care, was simply part of women's unpaid job.

The Metropolitan Borough of St Pancras certainly wanted women to clean up their environment. A booklet produced for their 1926 Health Week was filled with slogans like 'Where There's Dirt, there's Danger' and 'Now then, Mother, turn on the Tap, and get to work with the Soap'. There was no discussion of the housing and sanitation problems with which women might be trying to cope.

Councils ran Health Weeks to show women their 'Ideal Home', whilst failing to provide it in real life. A woman from Woolwich who lived with her husband and two children in one room wrote: 'I went to the Health Exhibition at the Town Hall, which I thought lovely especially the model houses.'

● Are women held responsible for making a safe environment today?

Women are still being told that their housing conditions are their own fault: 'When I told them my bathroom was damp they said well maybe your husband and your son miss the toilet when they pee.' (woman from a Liverpool housing estate) Other women have been told they shouldn't keep goldfish, or hang washing to dry inside.

Health education reinforces these ideas. The *Play It Safe* campaign, about stopping children's accidents, talks about keeping children away from cookers, paraffin stoves, and high windows, and taking them to safe playgrounds. It does not explain how you can manage this in a tiny kitchen, with children round your feet because there is nowhere for them to play, using a paraffin stove because it's the only heating you can afford. It does not mention that flats are often built with open-slatted staircases, swivel windows and unguarded balconies, and that playgrounds are often covered in tarmac and broken glass.

How much pressure is the Health Education Council putting on building designers, or on the Government to give more money for play facilities, compared with the pressure it is putting on women? The *Play It Safe* booklet is full of alarming, full-colour pictures of children with burns and scars, reinforced by phrases like:

'you can see that the scald is quite big and very sore.'

'you can see she burnt her bottom badly.'

This can increase the panic which women already feel, about how they can keep their children from harm in an unsafe world.

Maybe the Health Education Council will soon join with the Government's recent message to women (in TV advertisements and magazines) – to 'Keep the Under-Fives at Home' because the environment outside is so dangerous!

'How to manage your budget'

Health education was always concerned with teaching women to live economically. Child welfare classes concentrated on buying and preparing food on a limited budget. Typical titles of health education leaflets, written by well-off people, were 'How to Feed a Family of 5 on 12/9 a Week' and 'How to Spend 1/- on Food to the Best Advantage'.

The British Medical Association Committee on Nutrition criticised the working-class housewife for filling her family up with carbohydrates. A maternal mortality report accused women of 'ignorance of food values and unwise spending', because they bought fish and chips and tinned food. In fact, the 'ignorance' lay on the side of those who did not mention that it was very hard to get good fresh food in working-class areas. Also, women had little time to cook and few kitchen facilities, and cheap carbohydrates were often the only way to keep children from feeling hunger pangs.

Occasionally, patronising compliments were paid by the experts, who seemed surprised that women managed to feed their families without having had years of training in nutritional science. A member

...month we were almost ashamed to give recipes, ...y for very nice things, because of the industrial ...ich threatened so many of our homes with greater ...than usual. Fortunately the result was not so bad ...xpected, and for the miners' wives and families a ...spite is gained. Our sympathy goes out to the ...textile workers in their struggle. This month we ...o good family recipes, not too expensive and rather

Good Family Cake.

Ingredients

¾ lb. fresh roll (margarine).
½ lb. of brown sugar (foot sugar).
1¼ lbs. of flour.
½ lb. of seedless raisins.
2 eggs.
Pinch of salt.
2 tablespoonfuls of milk.

19 'Food Problems': page heading from *Labour Woman*, September 1925
At this time, the paper ran a cookery page with a difference – showing an
awareness of the difficulties women faced when planning their budget.

of the Medical Research Council referred to the mystery of the 'mar-
vellous instinct which seems to direct the purchases of food by so many
housewives', although he did accuse them of 'over-spending' at the
beginning of the week (presumably the only time when they could
spend at all).

Meanwhile, sample budgets in the Women's Health Enquiry
report showed reality – the incredible ingenuity that women used when
planning menus. One woman managed to feed three adults and one
child on 9/4d a week, mainly with soups and stews. In comparison, the
League of Nations 1935 'Diet for Mothers' would have cost 9/- or 10/- a
week for the woman alone. The average working-class wage at that
time was £2–£3 a week, and a large share of that had to go on rent.

Yet George Newman, in one of his yearly Ministry of Health
reports, said that malnutrition was 'due directly or indirectly to our
faulty habits and customs'.

• Is bad nutrition still considered to be women's fault?

Diets recommended by health workers often bear little relation to women's income. The National Council of One-Parent Families recently organised a survey of the diet sheets which London teaching hospitals gave out to pregnant women. At high-street prices, the diets cost around three-quarters of the money those women would have received on Supplementary Benefit.

Women have to shop for food which is cheap and filling:

'Baked beans and sliced bread – that's about all I can afford to stop them feeling hungry.'

'There's no point in telling us to cut down on meat. People on Social Security don't eat meat anyway – you can't afford it.'
(women keeping families on benefit)

Meanwhile, health education leaflets give the impression that women don't think carefully enough about diet. One leaflet on pregnancy says: 'This is a good time to think about what you eat and develop new eating habits, which will last . . . sensible eating will keep the family healthy.'

Although women today are faced with supermarkets full of food – is it healthy food? White bread and convenience foods, full of sugar and chemicals, cram the shelves, and are heavily advertised. Even 'fresh' fruit and vegetables may be weeks old and low in vitamins. Health education materials do not usually mention those problems.

The *How To Stay Alive* booklet dismisses the idea that chemicals added to food could be harmful. In a section on 'Allergies', additives are never mentioned as a possible cause, but plenty of space is given to telling women to breastfeed: 'Even one feed of cow's milk could start a newborn baby off with an allergic reaction . . . and multiply his chances of becoming allergic later in life.' So if your baby has problems, *you* are probably the guilty one.

• What is said about the diet of women from other countries living in Britain?

Asian and West Indian diets are usually much healthier than those of white British people. They contain the wholefoods (brown rice, kidney beans, lentils) which are a new idea to our supposedly advanced society. 'What did we used to eat in Jamaica? – rice and peas, fruit and vegetables. . . . Then we started getting other foods,

from America and Britain – you know, with lots of advertising.'
(British woman of Jamaican origin) Yet health education workers
often assume they need to convert the 'ethnic minorities' to
healthy eating.

For example, in this country there is little sunshine (which
helps our bodies to make Vitamin D) so we all need extra Vitamin
D in our diet. The Government makes sure Vitamin D is added to
margarine, but not to a food used by Asian people, such as chapati
flour. Instead, a special campaign has been mounted through
health education to convince Asian women to cook with margarine. Again, it is made to seem that black women, not Governments,
need re-educating.

Dying in childbirth – your own fault?

Women were also held partly responsible for the high maternal
mortality rate. The Committee which reported on this problem in 1932
listed four main reasons why women died in childbirth. One of these
was: neglect by the patient or her friends in making proper preparation
for the confinement (including refusal to follow medical advice).

Women were constantly accused of not going to ante-natal clinics
(although, in fact, reports showed that attendances increased greatly
during the 1930s – from 27 per cent of women giving birth in 1930 to 54
per cent in 1937). George Newman of the Ministry of Health thought
that it was 'strange and arresting' that women did not flock to ante-natal
clinics. Another medical expert, McCleary, also wondered why
pregnant women were 'slow to appreciate the advantages of ante-natal
care'. Perhaps the experts would have found the answer if they had
listened to a member of the Maternal Mortality Committee in
Manchester in the mid-1930s:

> 'We tried to get one [an ante-natal clinic] in Longsight and we had a
> petition. One reply came back saying there was no case because it was only
> 1.537 miles to walk. I remember saying well how would you like to walk
> 1.537 miles in the pouring rain.'

Newman even said that women were 'perhaps the greatest obstacle to
ante-natal care'!

Meanwhile, hardly any attention was focused on whether other
factors – such as poverty – might be responsible for the deaths of
women. In 1933, 1,291 official reports on maternal death reached the
Ministry of Health. Only twelve cases were said to be due to home

conditions and seventeen to malnutrition or physical weakness – but 298 were blamed on lack of co-operation by the patient!

A careful smokescreen was kept over the activities of doctors. Medical Officers of Health were reluctant to lay any blame on local colleagues. Newman also considered that if anything went wrong during the birth, it was largely women's fault. He stated that a woman 'ought to know better' than to cry for help during labour, since this might pressurise the doctor into hurrying and therefore causing an infection. (He did not mention that infections sometimes happened because doctors forgot to wash their hands before delivering babies, although this charge was often made against 'handywomen' who helped at births.)

In 1934, Edith Summerskill denounced the Ministry of Health's involvement with the medical profession. Until there was a woman Minister of Health, she said – and it should be a woman who had experienced a difficult labour herself – she did not think it likely that anyone would dare to criticise the dangerous practices of doctors.

● Are women still thought to be ignorant about pregnancy and childbirth?

Few women die in childbirth now. So even more emphasis than before is placed on the survival of the baby – and this is usually said to depend on the way pregnant women behave. The recent Government report on infant death, the Short Report, concludes:

> *'There is need to bring home to the public the very great importance and responsibility of childbearing, and the part they themselves play in ensuring the delivery of a normally formed and healthy child . . . this theme should be the foundation of all health education and Government policy.'*

Professor Oppé told this Committee that there should be 'a massive campaign to get mothers to be more educated in motherhood and to attend clinics and so on'.

Ante-natal clinics are still said to be one of the main aids to having a healthy baby, even though they often cannot solve problems which started because of poverty. One health education poster says of clinics 'there you'll be given all the special care and attention every expectant mother deserves.' Unfortunately, many clinics have changed little since the 1930s – yet women are still being criticised for not going to them.

The other main accusation against women now is that they damage their babies through smoking and drinking during pregnancy. Guilt-provoking health education posters hammer away:

'Do you want a cigarette more than you want your baby?'

'Is it fair to force your baby to smoke cigarettes?'

The stress of women's lives which often leads to smoking is not mentioned. Instead, the posters can add to the burdens women already carry, with terrifying warnings like: 'last year, in Britain alone, over 1,000 babies might not have died if their mothers had given up smoking when they were pregnant.' (Does 'might not' mean that other things – like poverty – *could* have been responsible too?)

It is often said that 'ethnic minority' women do not go to clinics often enough, and that this is the reason why their babies die more often than babies born to white women.

In fact, black women have, in general, worse housing, even more unhealthy jobs, and extra stresses including racism – all this must also affect pregnancy. At clinics they often meet racism too – being patronised or ignored. Health education campaigns rarely deal with these wider problems.

Conserving the traditional image of women

Health education reinforced women's responsibility to care for others and not for themselves. Government officials conveniently decided that this sense of duty was natural in women. Hilton Young, Minister of Health in 1934, said in Parliament: 'It is impossible and beyond the power of any man to prevent a mother sacrificing herself for the sake of her children.' More than twenty years earlier, the real truth had been pointed out by Anna Martin, who worked amongst women in Rotherhithe. She wrote in 1911:

'It is easier to attack the problem of infant mortality by founding Babies' Institutes, and by endeavouring to screw up to a still higher level the self-sacrifice and devotion of the normal working-class woman, than to incur the wrath of vested interests by insisting on healthy conditions for mothers and infants alike.'

It was made quite clear that a woman's job was to keep the family in working order, whilst asking the State for as little help as possible. The booklet produced by the Borough of St Pancras for their 1926

Is it fair to force your baby to smoke cigarettes?

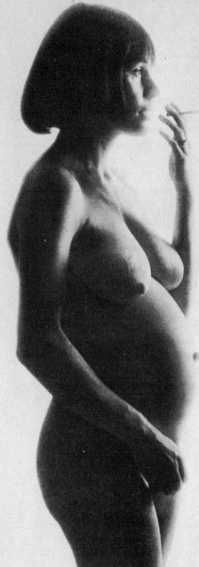

Is it fair that w̶ live in a society that forces us t̶ smoke cigarettes

Your b̶ through the umbilical co̶ bloodstream.

Smoking can restrict your baby's normal growth inside the womb.

It can make him underdeveloped and underweight at birth.

Which, in turn, can make him vulnerable to illness in the first delicate weeks of his life.

It can even kill him.

Last year, in Britain alone, over 1,000 babies might not have died if their mother had given up smoking when they were pregnant.

If you give up smoking when you're pregnant your baby will be as healthy as if you'd never smoked.

Turn over and find out how to stop.

20   Health education poster – as seen at the Women and Health Conference, 1981

Health Week began with the words 'Health is a Working Man's CAPITAL' and went on to explain that 'If a woman is ill, the home is neglected' – the man's capital would presumably depreciate rapidly. At times of national crisis, women were reminded even more strongly: the Food Economy Campaign Handbook, produced during the First World War, said 'The food problem remains: it is up to the women to solve it, and win the War.'

• Are women still encouraged to be self-sacrificing mothers?

A health education film on cervical cancer aims to persuade women to go for a cervical smear test, by showing a woman surrounded by her family: the commentary says that *they* need you to be fit. The title, *Think Of Us*, means that you should think of your husband and children – not that we should think of all the women who are at risk from cervical cancer.

Many health education campaigns have a lot in common with the advertisements that fill women's magazines, showing women working away at home for their families. They are like the well-known Flora margarine advertisement which tells you to 'look after your man' by making sure he's not eating too much fat. Women are supposed to watch out for the breadwinner, by counting the calories and the cholesterol.

Biological failures?

Even some enlightened campaigners for health agreed that women's central position in the family was natural and necessary. The Women's Health Enquiry report spoke of an 'abiding maternal personality' which made the woman 'the human anchor' of the family. The Peckham Health Centre, which was in many ways progressive and gave health care cheaply to working-class families, wanted to improve each woman's environment so that her 'instinct for wifehood and motherhood' would grow. They feared that, otherwise, families would become 'biologically deficient' and 'devitalised'.

A woman who was classified as an 'inadequate mother' was seen as a kind of biological failure. At a conference between the British Medical Association and the Ministry of Health in 1933, experts said that some women spent money unwisely and did not take enough care of their children, because of a 'broadly defeatist attitude towards life which has a physical basis' – as if problems were caused by a defect in the woman's body rather than by her stressful living conditions.

• Is motherhood seen as women's natural role by health educators today?

One Health Education Council pamphlet looks at 'What Does It Feel Like To Be A Mother?' Under the 'Wonderful' feelings you might have are:

> 'You . . . are now proven to be an adult, a Mother . . . you have joined the ranks of the special woman. You are one with Mother Nature, the Source of Life, the Madonna . . . you have reached the pinnacle of femininity.'

This reinforces the message women have heard since childhood – that true fulfilment only comes through motherhood.

The same pamphlet, *Now You're a Family*, lists 'Dreadful' feelings as well. Health education has become more sophisticated – it is now acknowledged that having a baby can make you feel 'exhaustion, resentment, depression . . . trapped'. But this is said to be 'normal'. You get the impression that eventually you will cope with everything – baby, housework, your husband's needs.

It is never suggested that the demands on women might be too much – that you might not want to be the only person looking after the baby, that your husband could share the housework, that you have a right to decent housing and a proper income. In fact, you are told to 'allow the other people (parents, husband, society in general) to have their feelings . . . but don't try to fight them.'

In another HEC booklet, you are told that if your own feelings are overwhelming 'you may be suffering from a mild depression. Tell your doctor in that case – it's a very treatable condition.' (Does this mean with Valium?)

• What is said about other ways of caring for children?

Many women come from cultures where babies are looked after by grandmothers, aunts, sisters, even fathers: 'You can leave your child with close relatives, a neighbour . . . the child is secure, we are so close.' (woman from Guyana)

But the nuclear family image is sold as 'progress' in Third World countries:

'In Bangladesh we hear that the right way to bring up children is in the European-style family, one father, one mother. When I came here I was surprised to find that people are not perfectly happy in these families, sometimes they are very unhappy.'

'It's much easier for the mother back home, here I have so much stress, no time to myself.' (woman from Bangladesh, and woman from Morocco, now living in Britain)

Why is the present-day British system of the isolated, anxious mother promoted as better, and other systems called 'inferior'?

● Have standards of motherhood changed since the 1930s?

Standards have, if anything, got higher. Motherhood has become a profession: you qualify for it by reading books on childcare, rather than learning from other women:

'Perhaps motherhood is the most important career for the majority of women, and yet today, while every other occupation demands a period of training, many mothers embark upon the most vital job of all without training of any kind.' (*Expectant Parents*, a leaflet from the National Association of Maternal and Child Welfare)

The experts now use psychology. In the first few weeks – even hours – of a baby's life, a woman must establish 'bonding' in order to be a successful mother. Breastfeeding campaigns emphasise 'bonding': 'Breastfeeding is better for your baby because it helps him to feel loved and secure.' Women who bottle-feed can end up feeling guilty, definitely not the Perfect Mother!

Women — the Race-Makers or Race-Breakers

Some people saw health education as part of the battle to make fit minds and fit bodies – so that the British nation could be dominant in the world. The National League for Health, Maternity and Child Welfare produced posters showing *How Mrs. John Bull Rears an A1 Family*. The People's League of Health was founded after the First World War to promote a 'Health Conscience and a Race Conscience' through health education, since, they said, 'Knowledge is the only armour of defence of which we cannot be robbed by an enemy.'

As in Nazi Germany, racial health was made out to depend on a special kind of discipline through which the body could become perfectly healthy. Part of this discipline required everyone to play their pre-destined biological role. So Oswald Mosley of the British Union of Fascists called for 'men who are men and women who are women', by which he meant that women must stay in their place as wives and mothers. Meanwhile, a major health education organisation, the Women's League of Health and Beauty, urged women to join well-disciplined exercise classes to improve their physique, since they were the 'Race-Makers or Race-Breakers'.

• Is racial health still a concern in health education today?

One of the latest ideas is 'pre-conceptual care' – getting health advice to women *before* they get pregnant. This sounds useful, but has worrying implications.

Women attending family planning clinics would be expected to discuss with their doctor whether they are fit enough to become pregnant. They would be told to cut down on smoking, eat a correct diet, and take more exercise.

Why is concern for women's health mainly shown when we might become pregnant? And why is it assumed that *all* women using contraception will soon want a baby?

Does the scheme have 'eugenic' implications: will black women and working-class women sometimes be advised not to have children?'

• For what other reasons does modern health education encourage us to look after our bodies?

Today, as well as being perfect mothers, women are also expected to make ourselves beautiful for men.

The booklet *Looking After Yourself* shows men wearing everyday clothes, playing football and jogging. Women are shown naked, posing seductively on the bathroom scales (checking their weight), or dancing sexily in tight shorts. Another booklet, *Stay Fit in the Office*, has cartoons showing women as sexy secretaries sitting on the bosses' laps, and the fitness being talked about is for the bosses, not the secretaries.

If women follow some HEC recommendations, they will not be fit – simply malnourished. The 'OK ideal weights' for women issued in the 1980 Look After Yourself campaign were so low that women who tried to reach that weight could find that their periods stopped (a sign of not eating enough), and they might be infertile. Why are we being told to slim so drastically?

Cigarette and drink advertisements make women worry about whether they are attractive enough. Health education campaigns use similar techniques to persuade women to *stop* smoking and drinking (for example, saying that if you smoke your mouth will taste like an ash-tray when a man kisses you). Such campaigns can further undermine women's self-confidence. Even if a woman gave up smoking, would her *overall* health have improved if she was doing it because she felt insecure about her sexuality?

Thus women are presented with confusing images in health education materials – the same images that we see in advertisements, in childrens' books, TV and magazines . . . glossy pictures of the perfect wife, happy mother, sexy call-girl, stupid female. None are realistic, but we are supposed to live up to all of them. Are materials like these really going to improve women's health?

Quiz

1 **You think your baby's got colic. Do you**

    (a) ask your doctor or health visitor for advice

    (b) ask your friend if her baby's had the same thing

    (c) ring your mother for advice?

Half the group answered (a) and half (c).

'You always ask your mother first anyway don't you.'

'With the first one I was on the phone every two minutes to my mum.'

'I thought my baby had colic for 12 weeks – but the doctor said breast-fed babies don't get colic.' ('Sounds like an old wives' tale to me,' said someone else in the group!)

Can books on bringing up children be helpful?

'It just comes natural – you don't need them.'

'I thought to be a good mother you had to read them, but they all contradicted each other.'

'There are some good books, but they should tell you, read this one.'

'The advice they give you at the hospital – they tell you to bath them night-time, well I found I had more time in the morning, night-time I'd be panicking . . . they ought to have a mum in there, a normal mum, to talk to the pregnant women, really they should.'

2 The 'Play It Safe' TV programme says 'keep kids away from busy roads'. Do you think

(a) I must be really careful with the kids

(b) but there isn't anywhere else for them to play

(c) there aren't enough lollipop ladies and zebra crossings?

Most people said (a) and a couple said (c).

'How can you keep them inside?' 'What do you do when you've got a lot of kids in a small place?'

'I can't stand those safety adverts.'

'That one with the kid drowning – it's horrible.'

'My little boy, he was crying in a corner after that advert had been on.'

'Maybe it shocks you into being a bit more careful.'

'But you worry all the time anyway.'

'You can be as careful as you like, because Trina, she was always after everything.'

'Every playground in the country is concrete.'

'That kid that fell off a balcony – they'd been on and on at the Council to make that balcony safe.'

'When you go to hospital with an accident with your kid, they treat you really badly, they treat you as though you've made it happen – and most people feel really bad about anything hurting their kids.'

'My boy slipped in the bath and got a black eye. I took him up to the hospital and they said, we're admitting him, he's got too many bruises – I said, do you think I'm mad enough to give him that last night and bring him up here today?'

'Yes, you have to really tell them at the hospital.'

3 You're told at the ante-natal clinic that if you don't eat properly your baby might not be healthy. Do you

    (a) think it's helpful advice

    (b) feel guilty that you're not eating properly

    (c) think the diet sheet's a bit hard to follow

    (d) wish you had more money to spend on food?

Most people said (a), one said (c) and several said (d).

'It's just common sense.' 'I wouldn't really worry about it.'

'Well before you're pregnant you might snatch something here and there, but once you're pregnant you think, God I've really got to think about it now, you make sure you have something a bit more nourishing.'

'I was so bloody sick I couldn't eat nothing anyway.'

The main issue seemed to be smoking in pregnancy:

'I felt guilty.' 'I felt terrible, I know it's bad for you.'

Why do women smoke?

'I had to really, I had to relax.'

'If a bloke's fed up he can walk out the door, you can't because of the kids, so you light up a cigarette.'

'I try not to stare at anyone when I see them smoking and they're pregnant, because I think sometimes it can even be a good thing if you need to relax.'

'I think it's terrible, the advertising, because most people are quite aware.'

'Because you smoke, it doesn't mean you think less of your baby.'

'If they don't want people to smoke they shouldn't sell them.'

'Times change, I mean this day and age women smoke, what will happen in the next day and age for women to do, it's always going to be put back to the woman.'

Do women get blamed directly for smoking?

'They induced me on the day he was due, because they said he was very small, and they said it was because I was smoking, and my husband said, I'm going to kill you, you should have given up – well he was there when David was born, David was 10 lb. 14 and he just couldn't say anything!'

4 Your doctor tells you to stop smoking because your chest is bad. Do you

(a) try hard to give up

(b) feel you can't give up because you need a cigarette to relax

(c) think there might be other reasons why your chest is bad, like the damp in your house, or the city air

(d) wish you had some real help in giving up?

Most people said (a). One said (b), a couple (c) and a couple (d).

What other factors, besides smoking, cause health problems?

'My doctor did tell me the pollution's really bad, that's why I had Laura there every two weeks with a cold.'

'They reckon this area's really bad for lead too.'

'Often you think, when you buy fruit off the market stalls and give it to the kids and you don't have a chance to wash it, you think, oh Christ I might have. . . .'

'Like all that about asbestos. . . .'

'They're getting big money out of it aren't they.'

'My friend lives on this estate in Battersea and she's saying the tenants are up in arms because it's in the central heating system.'

5 You see a leaflet on bringing up children. It's got a picture on the front, of a smiling mother with a baby, and her husband looking on. Do you think

(a) wish my family was like that

(b) looks very glossy – doesn't look much like me

(c) maybe if I read the leaflet I'll be able to be like that?

A couple of people said (a), several said (b) and one said (c). Comments written down were 'don't really take much notice, I like my family as it is', 'artificial' and 'looks nice – like many families I know'.

> 'Sometimes I feel that I wish my family was like that, sometimes you think Oh God, perhaps I ought to be. . . .'

> 'My breakfast-time, I'm shouting at my kids to sit down and shut up – in those pictures they're all sitting round in place all nicely turned out.'

Adverts in general were thought to be completely unrealistic:

> 'The setting for a start, all those beautiful houses.'

> 'That Imperial Leather advert, I mean can you imagine us all sitting in a big foam bath?'

> 'Like Persil, it doesn't really make everything white, only way I can do that is to use bleach.'

What's it really like at home with children all day?

> 'It's much easier actually to go out to work.'

> 'Why should you lose your identity, you're going to meet straight away women that have babies, you're going to talk about babies, you lose everything – when I took on this job I had no confidence in myself whatsoever and it was nothing to what I'd done before at work – it was just being at home for two years.'

> 'If you don't know where to turn for money, on Social Security, you don't know what to feed them on, I don't know how you'd cope.'

> 'I was really amazed a kid could get you so bad you'd want to slap them – when I used to read cases about battered babies I'd think oh my God how terrible, but I can understand it now, I can.'

6 A magazine article on slimming tells you the weight you should be for your height. Do you think

> (a) I'll start dieting again
>
> (b) that weight sounds very low to me
>
> (c) I like me the way I am
>
> (d) if I was slim I'd be more attractive?

Several said (b) and several (d). A couple said (c) and one said (a).

> *'I'll start my diet on Monday.'* (laughter)

> *'I keep on meaning to diet.' 'But if you did there'd be nothing left of you!'*

> *'I'd love to be slim but it is so hard for me – I don't care. Well I do care but I don't care. All our family are big though.'*

> *'If you're more of a motherly figure you don't get so many hassles.'*

Why do women often find themselves eating more?

> *'If you've got kids and not a lot of money coming in, and you're not happy with your housing, you might tend to eat, buy yourself a packet of biscuits for comfort.'*

> *'The more you try and diet, the more you eat.'*

Are women being pressurised to be slim?

> *'My husband says he'll leave me if I don't lose weight.'*

> *'My husband, no matter how much he goes on about it, I just ignore him, I say, I'll do it when I'm ready to do it.'*

> *'Why do you always get that on telly, the men have all got their clothes on and the women haven't?'*

Finally, we talked about spreading health information through women's health books and health groups.

> *'It might make you paranoid. Everything you hear about, you might think you've got it.'*

> *'I think they should tell you though, that if you're sterilised you might get depressed, because I got depressed and I didn't know why.'*

'It's good to hear about different people's views. Otherwise you start thinking you're the odd one out.'

'You might end up sounding like a lot of hypochondriacs.'

'I've got this friend, she's always got something wrong, it gets on my nerves.'

'There's always a few people like that though.'

'If you've got good friends maybe you don't need a group so much.'

'You don't get much time to talk though really, unless you're all at a playgroup meeting and you get off the subject.'

'Every Wednesday night we'll come round here then, have a night out!'

We looked at some books and pamphlets from the Women's Health Movement.

'All the headings in here sound interesting – I'd like to read about all these things.'

'Oh – that picture's definitely more realistic.'

One pamphlet quoted different women's experiences of breastfeeding:

'That's a good idea. They tell you breastfeeding's going to be wonderful but they don't tell you it can be agony with the baby hanging on to you as if you're a dummy!'

'Where can you get these books from?'

(For information about books and groups, see the end of this book.)

Suggested action

1 Ask older women, and women from different cultural backgrounds, about home remedies. For example, did your mother have a hand-written book of herbal remedies?

2 Find out if anyone has tried alternative forms of health care (acupuncture, herbalism, homeopathy, etc.). Are these

available locally? Can practitioners of these methods visit your group to explain what they do?

3 In a group which wants to learn more about health, make a list of topics to discuss. You can do your own research – from women's health books, from your own experiences. Maybe your group can write its own leaflets, make information posters about health, make a tape for a local radio programme, run a Health Day for women in your area.

4 Find out about local facilities for sports and physical activities for women. Would your local adult education institute run a course on women's self-defence or on relaxation and massage?

5 Get some frank opinions on what it's *really* like being a mother. How many women find it a pressure to 'keep up standards'? Is it common to feel angry with your children? Do you usually admit these things? or do you feel worried that you're the only one to feel that way? What kind of health education do you think would be useful for parents?

6 Collect pictures of women – in magazines, newspapers, etc. What are the common images of women in this society? Are they realistic? Do you like them? Find photos of yourself as a child, growing up, etc. How do you feel about these pictures? Were you/are you worried about your appearance?

Take photos of each other in everyday situations – washing up, going shopping with the children, at the factory or office, on holiday. How do these pictures differ from those in magazines?

If you wanted to draw cartoons about women's everyday lives, what would you draw?

7 Invent typical 'problem page' questions about health and relationships. What would your answers be?

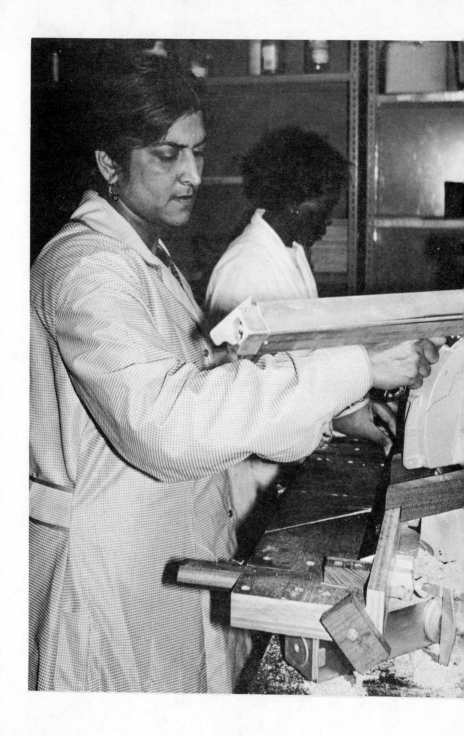

Chapter 5

HOW THINGS MIGHT BE CHANGED

Introduction: Where does women's strength lie?

Women have always been strong, coping with difficult conditions, managing to bring up families despite the odds. But is it to our advantage to keep on coping? Do we help our own health (or our families') by carrying on without protest? Is it time to look at our situation critically, and think of other ways of doing things?

Often women are too overworked to get round to complaining. We worry about joining unions or action groups, or even spending time talking to other women, because we don't want to neglect our families. We are frightened of making a stand about something in case things get even worse. Yet sometimes the burden of responsibility works the other way – the load becomes impossible, something snaps inside, and the feeling comes 'we've had enough, we can't cope unless we get better conditions'.

In the 1920s and 1930s, women joined together to demand better housing, higher unemployment benefit, more clinics. Once they took up a cause, they worked with great energy. They had an emotional commitment to their families from which they could not stand down.

At that time, women mainly saw themselves as wives and mothers, wanting to be able to look after their husbands and children better. Yet in order to work together, they had to assert themselves within their own homes too. This was often the most painful and difficult thing to do – but it led to feelings of independence. Today, many women are going one step further, saying that we deserve good health for ourselves as well, in our own right – trying to break away from the pressure which makes us see our lives only in terms of looking after other people.

The very strength which women summon up to survive can

Opposite: 21   Harsh Kalia cutting frames for jigsaws, Lambeth Toys Co-operative, September 1983
A group of women have organised this co-operative: they make their own decisions about work and wages, and have a creche for their children. Can other women's groups do the same?

work against us – if it keeps us quiet. But we can also use it *for* ourselves – we can draw on those powers of endurance in our struggle to be free.

This section examines what women have done, and are doing – in groups or as individuals – to make changes. It also looks at some of the things which stop us, including lack of confidence in ourselves.

Getting angry

Women's patience could not last for ever. Being told to be a good mother, whilst being forced to live in poverty, caused many outbursts like these:

> *'I am just about tired of bearing and nursing children. I have neither means nor time to do by them the justice I ought.'* (letter to Marie Stopes)

> *'If the State wants strong, healthy, useful citizens, they should provide the mothers in the homes with sufficient wages where the husband's wage is inadequate.'* (letter to the Women's Co-operative Guild)

Health education was sometimes given short shrift: the Maternal Mortality Committee in 1934 heard a typical story of a pregnant woman who was given a diet sheet at a welfare clinic and retorted, 'For goodness sake don't give me this! I want something to get food with!' At the 1936 Labour Women's Conference it was agreed that 'there is no wise way – from the point of view of health – of spending ten shillings a week for four people.'

• What makes women lose their patience today?

Again the first anger often comes because of the children. Here are some reasons women gave for forming tenants' action groups:

> *'We had really bad damp . . . we just couldn't bear to see our children suffer, and it was antibiotics, antibiotics, because they were always ill.'* (South Wales tenant)

> *'All the feelings of discontent came to a head after a child's accident. A toddler had climbed the balcony but leant too far out. I wondered how many would be interested in improving things by forming an Action Group, instead of grumbling in*

*groups on the way to the shops. The response was encouraging –
over 100 came to the first meetings.'* (Liverpool tenant)

Sometimes women simply refuse to 'manage' any longer. A
woman from Liverpool described what happened when a rent
strike began:

*'More and more women around here have stopped dashing off
to the moneylender in a sweat to borrow the money to pay off
their rent arrears. They're just saying "I can't afford two things
at once and I know which one's got to go!"'*

Better health for ourselves

Most women knew all too well where their ill-health came from:

*'Most of our incurable illness has been caused by the mother of the past
being underfed, and the horrid and heavy system of labour she has been
forced to live under.'* (miner's wife writing to the *Labour Woman*
newspaper, 1920)

*'I would not wish to have any more [children] as my health is not good,
through nothing but want of fresh air and more room which we can't get.'*
(letter to Marie Stopes)

As for welfare benefits, women grew tired of being expected to
manage without them. In 1921, the Ministry of Health suggested that
clinics should only provide meals for pregnant women on week-days,
missing out weekends: 'Are women to live like camels, getting suffi-
cient to carry them over the two days of scarcity?' asked the *Labour
Woman*. When the Minister withdrew this proposal, the paper commented 'apparently someone has told him that women are not camels!'

Those in powerful positions took the attitude that, as a contributor
to the *Labour Woman* put it, 'we are just poor women and there are
plenty more of us'. Not everyone was prepared to put up with being
treated like this. For example, some women writing to Marie Stopes
clearly thought they had a right to birth control:

*'as for the ministry of health they would rather learn us how to have them
rather than tell us how to avoid it.'*

*'all we get is looked down on treated like dirt where a little advice would do
a lot of good.'*

'the health visitor seemed disgusted with me when I asked her. I don't care

if I never see her again they are no good to us . . . they don't want us to
have birth control but thank god we have got it.'

• Do women feel strongly about facilities for themselves now as well?

Women's hospitals were set up many years ago – in the 1920s and 1930s women were glad of their existence, often finding them friendly and comfortable. Today these hospitals are still thought to be a good idea. When the Elizabeth Garrett Anderson hospital was threatened with closure in 1976, an occupation began, with staff continuing to work and keep the hospital open. They said:

> *'Elizabeth Garrett Anderson fought for this and I don't see why*
> *we shouldn't.'* (a shop steward)

> *'There are some things that women prefer to have treated by a*
> *woman.'* (a doctor)

In 1983, a similar campaign began, to save the South London Hospital for Women from closure.

Most women now see birth control as a basic right. When there was a proposal to close all the family planning clinics in East Sussex, local women in shopping centres were asked to sign petitions to protest. Without exception, women's reaction was complete disbelief: 'Close all our family planning clinics? They must be mad!'

Abortion, too, has finally become an issue that many women will talk about in public.

> *'The decision to have an abortion or have a child was something*
> *that only I could judge with any integrity. One of the things that*
> *appals me is that these issues are decided, not by the pregnant*
> *woman herself, whose body they are discussing, but by the*
> *politicians who pass the laws and the doctors who "assess" the*
> *situation, the majority of whom are men. My body is my own.'*
> (written by a woman after having an abortion)

• What happens when women have had enough?

Through their actions, women are saying that they feel differently about themselves. In the late 1970s, Asian women at several London factories went on strike against their working conditions.

> *'The manager started to shout at me, saying "Mrs. Desai, you can't talk back to me". . . . I said "I am here to tell you something but if you don't want to listen to me I am not going to listen to you either. . . . I am going to leave this job. . . . You misjudge people, you think they are daft. But they are not." '* (Grunwick factory worker)

A Liverpool woman described how she gained self-confidence when she became involved with a rent strike:

> *'I've always stood on the sidelines in the past, even on things like the closing of the wash-house. . . . I must admit I used to say "Oh, you can't win." But since my mate dragged me along with her to march with a lot of angry women to the Municipal Annexe on the rent increases, and seeing my own mates actually sitting on the floor and refusing to move and heckling – I've realised you've got to put up a fight for the things you need and want.'*

Getting together

The Women's Co-operative Guild provided many women with a chance to discuss common problems in a group. Members commented:

> *'I think if it had not been for the Women's Guild I should have been in the asylum.'*

> *'The testimonies of the health-giving properties of the Guild could almost rival those of Beecham's Pills.'*

Food prices, maternity services, abortion, housing problems – these were just a few of the issues dealt with by the Guild. The same themes were central to Women's Sections in the Labour Party, with their newspaper *Labour Woman*, and to women members of the National Unemployed Workers' Movement.

Women who had jobs outside the home were linked with those whose whole working day was spent in the home – through the Standing Joint Committee of Industrial Women's Organisations, which included the Co-operative Guild and Labour Party women, as well as the Women's Trade Union League.

• How are women organising today?

There are still many women involved in the Co-operative Movement, and in trade unions (two-thirds of new union members in the last twenty years have been women). Women's Sections of the Labour Party are now growing again. In Claimants' Unions, women have pressed for welfare benefits, and groups especially for women are starting up at Unemployed Centres.

Women's health groups meet informally to talk about all kinds of topics – menopause, tranquillisers, food and eating. . . . When there is a local problem about housing, road safety, or a clinic closing, a women's action group often starts up. Sometimes a campaign begins all over the country at once – like the National Abortion Campaign when there was a threat to change the Abortion Act in 1975.

Women health workers (nurses, midwives, health visitors and doctors) are forming their own radical organisations. They would like to create a health service which is sympathetic to women, and in which different health skills are shared out or equally respected, so that the present hierarchy is challenged and changed.

Making new ideas

Women wanted to learn more – not from people in authority, but from each other and from people they could trust. They entered into energetic discussion of the problems which needed solving.

Sometimes knowledge was passed on in secret. A woman who often spoke to meetings in working-class areas reported that abortion help was 'the only talk among women . . . they're very loyal together, and what one knows goes all up the street.'

Other matters could be discussed more openly. Labour Party Women's Sections ran talks on housing, which emphasised the effects of darkness and damp on health, and said that rest homes for TB were a waste of time when the cause of the illness was not being tackled. When looking at nutrition, Labour women learned new information, like the need for vitamins – at the same time, they discussed the fact that welfare benefits were too low to provide a healthy diet.

Education happened in many different places. Inexpensive pamphlets were read by women in their own homes. Sometimes meetings were organised out on the street, such as in the Bethnal Green 'Women's Revolt' of 1928, when subjects included the following: the need for higher benefits, free boots for women and children, the possibility of setting up their own baby clinic. Women who began going out to their local branch of the Labour Party or the Co-operative Guild sometimes went even further afield: to week-long summer schools or national conferences. A *Women and Unemployment* conference in Scotland in 1935 lasted two days – housing, rents, and the dangers of childbirth were important topics.

In these meetings women looked at the reasons which made their lives so difficult – to find out what was causing their problems. In 1933, Labour women found that although they were suffering a shortage of milk, Britain actually had a milk glut! The farms were selling lots of milk to manufacturers at 1½–2½ pence a quart (the price in the shops was around 6d.).

• What kind of discussion about health goes on amongst women today?

Probably more women set up groups now especially to talk about health. Often these groups would see themselves as part of the Women's Health Movement, which is not an organisation with official members – it is a huge informal network of women everywhere who are working for change. The link between the groups is the belief that we have a right to a society which is healthy for everybody, which gives good-quality health care, and in which women can lead their own lives.

'Self-help groups' can start in many ways. One woman in South London felt depressed after a hysterectomy operation. She wrote a simple leaflet saying 'Come for coffee and a chat' and it was given to women as they left hospital after the operation. Other women have put notices in shop windows or community centres. Throughout the country, women's health courses are run – through adult education, for mother and toddler groups, in youth centres.

Once women get together, they often discover they are not alone, and they can help each other.

'Eight of us sat around and talked about PMT [pre-menstrual tension], and it was so helpful just to get it real in your heads, just to say oh you've got that as well, have you tried such and such a thing or oh god, dropped fifteen milk bottles today.'

You can also look for the reasons behind common problems.

One Family Health Group wrote a pamphlet called *Scream*: this is how they explained the name:

'Initially we met to talk about children's health/illnesses. However, it soon emerged that our most pressing problems stemmed from our limited roles as "Housewives". What came up time and time again was the frustration women at home with children face.'

Some issues, such as bad housing and hazards at work, are more often worked on by Labour parties and trade union branches (and women's action groups – see pp. 127–30). Trade unions run courses on health and safety, some especially for women, so that safety representatives know about the dangers of chemicals and shiftwork, for example.

Arguing on our own terms

Sometimes women entered into a debate with official organisations, armed with their own facts. In 1933, Labour women challenged the British Medical Association's 'minimum diet', on which a working-class family was expected to be able to survive. Labour Party Women's Sections asked their members to write down their own weekly budgets and say what they thought of the official one.

It became obvious that the BMA diet was ridiculous: for example, the prices referred to were completely wrong (much lower than actual prices in local shops), some items were almost impossible to buy in working-class areas (such as cow's milk), some obvious foods had been completely left out (such as eggs). Everyone thought the BMA diet was 'dreary' – they were much more imaginative themselves on a tiny budget – and some of the amounts in the recipes were quite wrong! And the oddest thing of all: 'Imagine a mother trying to spread ½lb. of butter and ½ lb. of margarine on 39½ lb. of bread!'

- **Are women still insisting on using our own evidence?**

In 1976 many progressive organisations boycotted a Select Committee on Abortion, which had been set up by Parliament to look at possible 'abuses' of the Abortion Act. The Committee was mostly made up of male MPs opposed to abortion.

Instead of giving evidence to this anti-woman group, the

campaign for a woman's right to choose about abortion decided to put *them* on trial – along with those doctors, churchmen, and Department of Health officials who were denying abortion facilities to women – to point out that these were the people who really abused the law.

Two thousand people met in London in January 1977 for the Abortion Rights Tribunal. Local groups of the National Abortion Campaign (NAC), health workers and individual women spoke out to say that facilities must be extended, not cut back. Birmingham NAC's evidence said:

> *'In Birmingham it's three times more difficult to get an abortion than in Newcastle. . . . Dr McLaren [an anti-abortionist] is the chief gynaecologist. . . . Working-class women already have to run the gauntlet to get what is supposed to be theirs by right under the 1967 Act.'*

Changing the plans

Often women drew up alternative plans and tried to get the authorities to listen to them. For example, in 1917, a pamphlet called 'The Working Woman's House' was circulated round Women's Sections of the Labour Party. Members were asked to comment on two different plans for a simple cottage.

By June 1918, forty-five local conferences had been held on the subject. The following things were generally thought to be important: a separate bathroom with bath; a well-equipped scullery kitchen with gas stove and hot water; a wide front to the house to let in plenty of sunlight.

The Government made a show of being interested in working-class women's ideas, by inviting their organisations to send representatives to a new Housing Council in 1919. By 1920 the women had decided that the Council was 'an entire farce' – since it had not met for a year! As a Scottish miner's wife put it when she was trying to get on to a local housing committee, the officials were 'not very anxious to be stirred up'.

Similarly, the Women's Co-operative Guild had detailed plans for a national maternity service – including more women doctors, more household helps, and a longer period of maternity benefit. All the women's organisations wanted a State maternity service, so that they were not forced to depend on unsympathetic insurance societies for their health care. They saw this as a right.

PLAN OF HOUSE.

GROUND FLOOR.

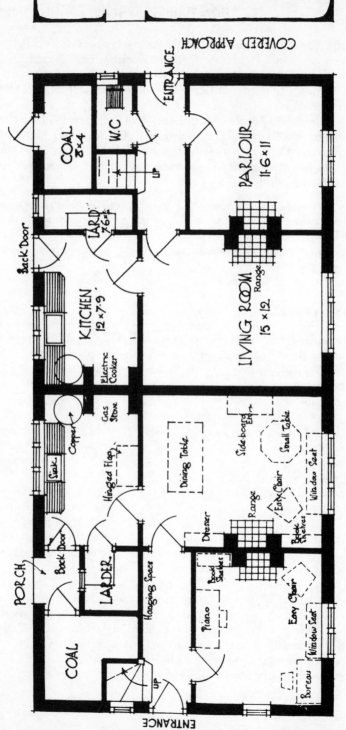

These houses would be placed in blocks of four, with a small space of grass in front. The groups might be arranged in many ways—round quadrangles, in tree-

Between each set of two houses would be a covered approach, and over this a sleeping-out balcony (especially valuable for delicate or tubercular people) could be

They were definitely looking for good-*quality* care. A nationwide survey amongst Labour women showed a very low opinion of ante-natal clinics. Although women thought ante-natal care was a good idea, their criticisms included: clinics were too far away – they couldn't afford the transport to get there; the atmosphere was depressing and uncomfortable; they had to wait for hours; the doctors seemed to think 'working women don't know the meaning of words.' (Do these criticisms by any chance sound familiar?) The report ended by saying – was it surprising that women did not always attend clinics?

Where even basic facilities were not available, women stated clearly that they wanted them. In 1934, the Wolverhampton Guilds tried to get a clinic set up, with a woman doctor, for women over forty, since at this age women had extra mental strain and fears of cancer. Some women's organisations also made radical demands about abortion. For example, in 1934 the Women's Co-operative Guild passed a resolution:

> *'This Congress calls upon the Government to revise the abortion laws of 1861 by bringing them into harmony with modern conditions and ideas, thereby making of abortion a legal operation which can be carried out under the same conditions as any other surgical operation.'* (Only fifteen women out of 1,360 voted against this.)

- ## Are women suggesting alternatives now?

Some tenants' groups have pressed hard to be involved in decisions about their housing. One group managed to arrange meetings with housing officials, and a woman who went said

> *'What a cheek I appeared to have, telling them where they had gone wrong. They with their huge salaries and diplomas and years of "experience" . . . they didn't like it when I told them the only way they could understand just how bad Netherley was would be by living there themselves.'*

She went on:

> *'We wanted to change the allocations procedure . . . we went round conducting surveys, collecting cuttings from newspapers. I read all I could get my hands on about housing. Finally we prepared a report.'*

Opposite: 22   Plans for 'The Working Woman's House', 1918
Labour Party Women's Sections gave their views on this plan. Two alternative suggestions are shown here for the ground floor. The plans are exact and detailed, drawn up by women themselves, based on practical experience from their daily work at home.

The Council did pass some new proposals, although the group didn't think they went far enough.

Another tenants' group, in London, found out that there were asbestos panels in the walls of their flats. They arranged a public meeting to give tenants information about asbestos hazards. An Asbestos Action Group was formed to talk to Lambeth Council and demand that the asbestos be removed. After a few months the Council agreed to do this.

Women are constantly agitating for more health services and better ones. In Stockwell, South London, a group met together when they heard that a new health centre was to be built locally. They consulted sympathetic women architects and made suggestions for the design of the Centre, including a community café, and space for counselling and community groups. These plans went to health service administrators, who agreed to include local people in future discussions. Hopefully, Mawbey Brough really will be 'a health centre for the community'.

Making our own arrangements

Occasionally women were able to set up practical services for themselves, in connection with health. In some places, fund-raising activities were held to provide extra money for women when they were pregnant. In one industrial area, women had a secret 'abortion club' – they paid in a weekly sum to build up a fund, to pay for abortions, and to pay for travelling to another town to get one if necessary.

Another issue on which women had some kind of alternative was in buying food and goods for the family. They could shop at Co-operative stores, which tried to keep prices reasonable, gave a share of the profits to members, and only sold goods which had been made in trade-union-organised workplaces, where the workers got a decent wage. The Women's Co-operative Guild appealed to the power of 'the woman with the basket' – it was a limited way of trying to affect the economy, but it had possibilities.

• Have women started up new services recently?

A group in Rochdale decided they wanted a Well Woman Clinic, where women could talk about any health problem and find out how to stay healthy.

'The first big thing that we did was to hold a public meeting in Rochdale Town Hall, and two hundred women turned up. One of the people from the Area Health Authority was there, that was the meeting that changed his mind. Everyone wrote their name down who wanted to be involved . . . the campaign was under the umbrella of the Community Health Council. We talked to every women's group and women's club, anything to do with women in the Rochdale area, asking them what sort of clinic they would like.'

Running health courses was a way of getting more women involved: 'We ran two courses for six weeks, one evening each week . . . they were very well attended and we got a lot more support for the campaign.'

They put their case to the Area Health Authority, who agreed that a clinic could be started, although they wouldn't give money for a doctor at first. This turned out to be an advantage in some ways!

'We were given a disused clinic – we run every Tuesday from 5 to 9 with volunteers. We're from different backgrounds, some of us are health visitors, some have counselling experience, some of us know a bit more about nutrition. We're beginning to know our own strengths. One woman, who didn't feel confident enough to counsel people, she's beginning to say "Perhaps one day I'll do a bit of counselling".'

What happens when someone arrives at the clinic?

'She's welcomed in, offered a cup of tea and the chance to sit down and chat. We've found that a lot of women can be helped just by talking to us. We have a questionnaire, it's really intended to have the woman look at it for herself, she might say "oh well I've never thought about that" – like how many people have you got at home, and have you been feeling tired lately, and what did you eat yesterday. Not everybody does the questionnaire, some people already know exactly why they've come.'

All the clinic workers are equal:

'We don't treat the health visitors separately, they roam around the same as everyone else, making cups of tea . . . we don't wear any labels. If I was counselling a woman on contraception, I would go and get another woman at the clinic who knows a lot about it, she's not a health visitor. Some of the health visitors

who normally would say "you need a doctor" are trying to break out of that mould.'

Can the clinic help women to get over problems without using drugs? 'Sometimes it's the woman's nutrition that's at fault. Sometimes women need extra vitamins. For example, Vitamin B6, some women need a lot at a certain time.' What happens when women go back to their doctors?

'With a lot of people we say, look you will have to go back to your own doctor, but come back and tell us how you get on. Some women have come back and said, my doctor was much better when I went back because I had more information and I was more confident, I could ask him more questions and he could see that I wanted to know.'

This conversation was recorded when two women from the Rochdale Clinic were talking to members of other Well Woman Clinic campaigns. There are about eight such groups in the Manchester area – some have managed to get a clinic too. The groups meet regularly to get ideas and help from each other.

Another project run by women is an Asian Food Co-operative in Stonebridge, North West London. It began when an Asian Women's Group talked about making jobs for themselves. Six women work in the Co-op, cooking Asian food and selling it to local restaurants and factories. They are providing healthy food, which for most people is hard to come by, and they also have more control over the conditions in which they work.

Face to face with the authorities

Sometimes the opportunity came up to speak directly to people in power – either through invitation, or by arriving and demanding to be heard. Women made the most of these occasions.

In 1919 the Coal Industry Commission heard evidence from mine-owners, saying that miners' wives were unclean and were bad cooks. Several miners' wives were invited to the Commission and given right of reply. The women gave graphic descriptions of the conditions in which they lived. As they said, it might be necessary to clean the house four times a day as the men came home from each shift – it was a miracle that miners' houses were kept so spotless. As for the accusation that miners' wives kept coal and chickens in the bath, one woman explained that this was a practical answer when baths were put in such inconvenient places (in tiny sculleries with no water) – it was much easier to carry on bathing in a tub by the fire!

In East London towards the end of the First World War, a group of women went uninvited to see Lord Devonport, the Government representative in charge of food supplies. They were tired of standing for hours in queues to get bread or potatoes. Lord Devonport became 'very excited', reported the *Woman's Dreadnought* newspaper, when he heard that the women thought all food shops should be taken over by the Government. With rather the same attitude as Marie Antoinette, he asked, 'Why can't you get bread? Is there more bread eaten than there used to be?'

The women told him in strong words that they could not get potatoes, thus everyone wanted bread and there was not enough. Lord Devonport became 'uncomfortable', especially when the women told him they didn't want to be offered any more fancy cakes – the sugar made them feel sick because they were so unused to it.

• Can you go directly to 'the top' to say what you think?

After talking about nutrition at a Women's Health Course, some women from Wigan decided that something needed to be done about school dinners.

> *'We live in a very very poor deprived area, we've nothing in Platt Bridge, nothing . . . we've just done a campaign for our children's school dinners, we worked very hard, that was just through this Women and Health course, give us confidence for it. . . . They kept saying we've no money, but guess what, I told her as if she didn't put better meals on . . . this was the head of the Education Meals Department and I said, they're not starving my son, look I've had six kids and five have gone through that school and they've the worst dinners. . . . So we wrote to Margaret Thatcher, we wrote to everybody, and guess what? they have a two-course choice now, fantastic dinners. They weren't getting fed before.'*

Frustration – and direct action

Sometimes, after trying for a long time to make the authorities listen, women decided to make their point more forcefully. They were tired of being ignored.

At the Maternal Mortality Committee meeting in 1928, the Minister of Health urged 'courage and patience'. One woman asked how he could expect patience when her local area wanted to build a maternity centre but couldn't get the Ministry's permission to use land for it? In 1932, a Co-operative Guild representative spoke out at the same annual gathering, saying that she had been going to these meetings for fifteen years and now she wanted the conference to 'come down to rock bottom and do something that will have some result'.

It was not surprising that women sometimes wanted to shout out loud. In 1934, a healthy young woman died after childbirth: she had had her baby in the out-patients' department of a Manchester hospital because there was no bed for her. Hundreds of angry women came to a public inquiry about her death.

One way of pointing out the shortcomings of welfare facilities was for everyone to claim their rights at once. In the early 1920s, people were often told that they were not going to get any more benefit – they had to manage without, or go to the workhouse (the authorities bargained on people being too ashamed to do that). But in Battersea in 1921, a thousand people (including many pregnant women) marched on the workhouse together, demanding to be housed. Of course the workhouse could not cope. Seven hundred people – women, men and children – stayed all night to make their protest. Several women actually gave birth there. The marchers insisted on receiving decent food, and instead of the usual 'disgusting' meals, they were given roast beef and potatoes.

Such protests showed that large numbers of people were angry. By coming together, people felt the support of others, and gained more strength to carry on their fight. The newspaper *Out of Work* described the Battersea marchers: 'Not a head dropped, all held high, all realising the dignity of their position, and strong in their determination.'

Women were always present. On the 1932 Hunger March, the women's contingent marched from Burnley to London. Ellen Wilkinson, a Labour MP, saw 'those indomitable middle-aged women who are the backbone of local Labour Parties' on the famous Jarrow marches.

Women also stood out bravely in strikes. In 1932 the Lucas engineering firm started to speed up production lines. Many of the young women workers collapsed from extra strain. Finally they went on strike, refusing the new system – for eight days, they stayed inside the factory, singing protest songs and shouting when the management came 'Throw them through the window.' Alarmed, the firm gave in.

Women sometimes threatened to take what was not being given to them. During the bread and potato shortage in London in 1917, angry crowds of women collected outside fish and chip shops, ready to break in – until the police had to set up a sale of potatoes to them.

● What kinds of direct action have women tried recently?

Bureaucracies still frustrate women who want to get something changed. 'The public can go once a month to the Area Health Authority meeting, but you've not to speak!' (Well Woman Clinic campaigner) A shop steward at the Elizabeth Garrett Anderson Hospital explained why the staff finally decided to occupy the building: 'It has been an extraordinary process. . . . It's come as a last resort – we've been through everything and just been kicked.'

This was not the only hospital to be occupied by people who wanted to keep it open. Hounslow Hospital, Bethnal Green, Plaistow Maternity, St Benedict's . . . these are a few out of many others. Support always came from local people:

'The pensioners' club came to protest at the Area Health Authority, and they were terrific, singing and dancing and they all had banners. Someone lifted one lady up to the office windows and she was banging on them and saying "Come out here, you miserable old gits!"' ' (Save Bethnal Green Hospital campaigner)

A South Wales tenants' group also found that dramatic action was the only way to get heard.

'We started in the usual way, with petitions and writing letters and we were more or less ignored and called educationally sub-normal. One of us said "what we ought to do is to chain ourselves to the bloody railings" and the next thing is, we did it! It was incredible. The press were coming, the television were coming. Suddenly even our councillors greeted us.'

An Action Group in Kent started when three women decided that a dangerous road needed a pedestrian crossing. They got no reply to their letters, so they organised demonstrations and blocked the road completely. Finally the county councillors agreed to take the matter up. Meanwhile, the same group managed to have a playing field fenced to stop children running into the road, and they got their street lights turned back on when the Council turned them off to save money.

Two women in South London organised a street group to try to get rubbish cleared out of their area. One woman began collecting the rats – and delivering them alive to the Council!

Women in paid work have often resorted to strikes over health issues. Five women cleaners at a London polytechnic began coughing as they swept up asbestos dust which covered the floor 'like a lot of snow'. They refused to work again until the building was cleared up by specialist cleaners who had proper protection.

At Grunwick's factory in North London, Chix sweet factory in Slough, and Futters factory in Brent, Asian women were the mainstay of the picket line, on strike to get better pay and healthier working conditions. They refused to be intimidated by violence: at Grunwick's, two women were run down at the factory gate by a driver who was breaking the strike; and when huge numbers of sympathetic people came to make a mass picket, the police tried to break the crowd up.

In 1982, health workers all over Britain, many of them women, went on strike for higher wages, and for the NHS to have more money so that it can provide better care.

Women were also present on the 1981 People's March for Jobs. Women's contingents walked from Liverpool, Wales and Yorkshire to London. Some marchers wore sashes saying 'a woman's right to work' – to say that women need paid jobs as much as men do.

What holds us back?

We need to look at the things which *stop* women from making changes. There are so many pressures coming from outside us and inside us: we need to know what these are and decide what to do about them.

The opinions of men

Men in authority did not appreciate women being outspoken! One way to put women down was to label them as ridiculous. In 1936, when a deputation of Welsh women went to request a better maternity hospital, the Medical Officer of Health described this as 'wild, hysterical effusions by the women of Llanelly'.

Even working-class men were usually far more interested in having women look after them, than in their wives becoming involved in campaigns for better living conditions. In the short term, it was more pleasant to be welcomed home with a meal. Hannah Mitchell, busy all her life campaigning for votes for women, said that there was no escape from 'the tyranny of meals'. She noted that there was much talk about 'comradeship' between men and women, but 'these Socialist young men expected Sunday dinners and huge teas . . . exactly like their reactionary fellows.'

In 1939, the *Labour Woman* printed a lively play, *Sarah Sees It Through*, for local Women's Sections. Bob (Sarah's husband) and Jim (Ellen's husband) come back to find their homes empty – no Sarah, no Ellen. But they *do* find a leaflet:

> *Jim* (reads it out) 'Special meeting for women to be held in Co-op Hall'. . . . Ellen hasn't gone there, she knows I object to women bothering in politics.
> (Enter Ellen and Sarah)
> *Jim* Have you been to this meeting?
> *Ellen* Ay.
> *Bob* Women's place is at home.
> *Sarah* Oh is it? Well if home's such a grand shop as all that, why don't you stop home more than what you do?
> *Jim* We've been working and we need a change.
> *Sarah* Well haven't we been working in the house all day? It's just us as *should* go out for a change. . . . It's time you changed your ideas, trying to make your homes into prisons for your wives.
> *Jim* By gum! If this is what happens after going *once* to a meeting, we'll know what to expect. . . .
> (But Sarah and Ellen continue their political activity and insist on having more freedom.)

● What is men's reaction to women getting involved in things today?

Women are often treated in a patronising way when they are angry about something. A South Wales tenant said: 'Whenever we met officials they would try and put us down. . . . We met this by screaming, shouting and going hysterical in public. They didn't know how to handle it.' So sometimes it seems the only option is for women to become hysterical!

Husbands often object to women's action. The Asian women on strike at Grunwick's decided to talk to their husbands as a group.

One Sunday, forty of them met together with their husbands, to explain why the picket line was vital.

Sometimes men change their attitudes to their wives when action happens: 'My husband has respected me a lot since then,' commented a woman who became involved in a housing group. Other men feel threatened: 'He says "Good God, you're not the same woman as you were a year ago. You don't fetch and carry like you used to." ' (member of Welsh tenants' association)

Health is women's responsibility

Many organisers of progressive political groups also thought women's place was at home – the difference was that they wanted women to *improve* their homes, by campaigning about housing and food policies. Men were busy on pay and problems at work. The caring role was once again left to women.

Marion Phillips, Labour Party Women's Officer, wrote:

'There are certain matters in which the experience of women is wider than that of men can ever be; those matters . . . which most intimately concern home life, the nurture of the young, the care of the sick and weakly, the planning of the dwelling.'

She seemed to think that this was a biological fact, rather than that it could be because women spent all their time at home – and she did not suggest that men should start to develop their experience by doing housework or looking after children.

A Labour Party pamphlet on housing began 'Woman's chief task is to make a home.' Ethel Bentham of the Party Executive wrote to the *Labour Woman* about 'women's responsibility for the health of the State'.

A woman member of the National Unemployed Workers' Movement commented that 'anything peculiar to women is left over' – including such vital issues as food centres, clinics, and maternity homes. The Women's Sections were expected to deal with all of these.

During the 1926 miners' strike, it was women who distributed food and clothing to strikers' families. A. J. Cook, a prominent Labour man, praised Labour women for 'caring for humanity'.

Strikes meant extra work for women. It was harder to manage when even less money was coming in – but they were still expected to cope somehow. Men's vision sometimes seemed to stop short at the workplace; campaigns for higher wages were the be-all and end-all.

WOMEN VOTE LABOUR

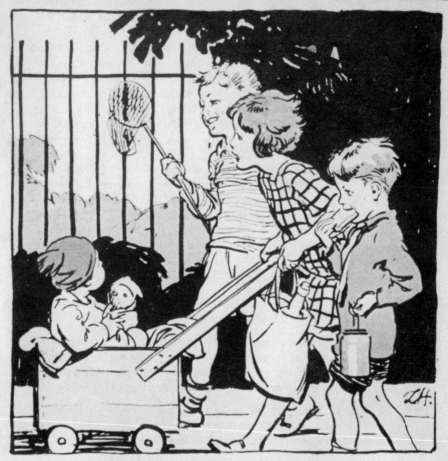

FOR THE CHILDREN'S SAKE

23 'Women Vote Labour': Labour Party poster, 1928
Why were women being urged to vote for their children's sake rather than
for their own?

Labour Party women in South Wales went to the Miners' Federation in 1920, asking them to fight for lower prices *as well as* higher wages.

So in some ways women had a fuller understanding of politics than men – the politics of living and surviving, eating and keeping warm. Women were often the backbone of strikes, despite the difficulties caused for them, because they knew – even more than the men – how desperately they needed to win.

Sometimes women insisted on continuing when the men wanted to give in. As one woman in a mining village said, 'We are prepared to support our men if only they will make a kick against having to live in the hell we are in today.' In 1927 in Durham 'an army of enraged women' came to tell union officials that they were 'near to breaking point'. They felt the officials were not fighting hard enough on the strikers' behalf. 'They may kid the men for a little while – but they don't kid the women.'

If a strike failed, women sometimes felt betrayed. They were divided from men in their opinions, because they had struggled alone to provide for the home. If men and women had been equally responsible for home and for the work outside it, would they have felt more united in times of difficulty?

● Do women still deal mainly with welfare issues?

Often women start to do something about a health problem because they live with it all the time.

> *'It's got to be women, we're the only ones that can understand the problem. The men are out all day. My husband would never have done anything about it. He didn't have to sit there with the rats running over his feet.'* (housing campaigner)

> *'I think it's because the men couldn't care where they go, it's the women that have to bring the children [to hospital] and things like that.'* (woman from campaign to save a hospital)

So men don't get involved because they don't take responsibility for the home in general. A woman who helped to organise a rent strike was bitter that many men told their wives that a strike wasn't necessary. 'Once the men hand the money over that's their responsibility finished, isn't it? And if anything happens when you haven't paid, it'll all fall on you, won't it?'

Is it good that these matters are left to women – or is it a burden? Do we want men to take an equal part in working for better health care and housing? If so, it looks as though we'll have to get them to share the work at home – so that they can see what the problems really are.

Taking care of the Party

As well as looking after their homes, Labour women also had to look after the Party. At election time, women conscientiously went canvassing. (Hannah Mitchell said that, in her experience, men often sat drinking cups of tea.) Marion Phillips said about election work: 'It seems unreasonable and unsympathetic to press it so upon women who are already overworked. But we have to do it because it is the only way to accomplish Labour's triumph at the elections.'

In the Unemployed Movement, sewing classes were arranged during which women could 'discuss the problems of the day' whilst simultaneously making banners for marches! As always, women were expected to do two things at once.

It was not clear whether men in the organisations really wanted women to be free – or just to be wiser wives and mothers. The newspaper *Out of Work* described their ideal woman on a march: 'that heroic woman, hatless, red-faced, baby at breast, panting to keep up with her man'. Another issue of the paper carried 'A Word to Unemployed Women'. It said: 'You are the producers of humanity. Join your men-folk, if only out of respect for the kiddies that will follow you.'

If women wanted changes for themselves – for example, if they wanted to stop producing humanity – they got a strong reaction. From 1924 onwards, Labour Party Women's Conferences voted unanimously for the State to provide birth control facilities for all women. The subject aroused a lot of excitement amongst women. Yet Party leaders remained strongly against birth control. One Labour woman said, at an International Women's Conference, 'If our men had known birth control was going to be discussed, they would not have let us come.'

The *Labour Woman* newspaper said in 1918: 'Labour stands for no sex in politics. It demands equality', and an 'appeal for unity at home' in the same issue asked men and women to 'look their differences fairly and squarely in the face and see whether they are not imaginary'.

Women who wanted birth control, equal rights to jobs, and help with the housework were not seeking the kind of equality the Labour Party leaders had in mind.

● **What is the attitude towards women in progressive organisations today?**

Women are making their presence felt in the Labour Party, in trade unions and in many similar organisations. But there is still a long way to go. For example, the TUC backed the huge demonstration for abortion rights in 1980, but didn't want women to lead the march!

Although the last Labour Government passed laws on equal pay and maternity pay, and against sex discrimination, there are very few women in powerful positions in the Labour Party. But many women in Labour Party Women's Sections want real equality, which means sharing the work *inside* the home as well as sharing the jobs outside the home. Many calls are made to women to be active trade unionists – but are trade union leaders calling on their male members to be active in doing the housework? Why is a very basic right, a woman's right to control her own fertility, still being held back? Officially, the Labour Party says that any woman who wants an abortion should be able to get one on request, but whenever there is a vote about abortion law in the House of Commons, MPs are left 'free to vote according to their consciences'.

A recent headline in a local Labour Party paper says 'Labour Women Make Policy Not Tea!' If the women who campaigned in the 1920s and 1930s could see that headline, they would probably identify with it too!

24 'Call a meeting on women after work and what happens?': cartoon
It is often said that women aren't interested in union meetings. Is this really the case?

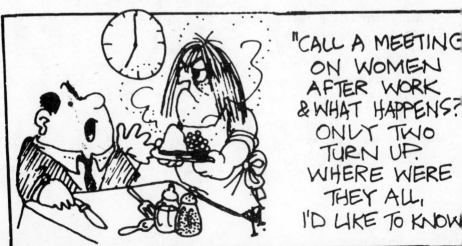

"CALL A MEETING ON WOMEN AFTER WORK & WHAT HAPPENS? ONLY TWO TURN UP. WHERE WERE THEY ALL, I'D LIKE TO KNOW

Lack of time

Women often found it difficult to concentrate on new activities – children, housework, and other people's needs not only took up time, they also took up space in each woman's mind. As one woman wrote to the Co-operative Guild in 1915: 'I am afraid I cannot tell you much because I worked too hard to think about how we lived.' Another woman found it hard to write a clear account of her life to Marie Stopes; she finished, 'please do try and bear with me as baby is crying.'

Even when they managed to get involved in action, women were limited by their home responsibilities. The *Woman's Dreadnought* newspaper described how women at a lively meeting about food prices suddenly heard the twelve o'clock horn sounding from the docks. Instantly they were reminded that they were wives and mothers, and they scattered home in all directions.

● **Do women feel distracted in the same way today?**

A woman who became an active member of her Tenants' Association wrote:

> *'Up to a couple of years ago, the children were my LIFE. If I left Roy with anyone so that I could go out I'd be thinking all the time "are the windows safely locked where he is?" When a man goes away from home and from the kids, he forgets. He puts them out of his mind.'*

Does it help women to worry so much about other people? Could we try to free our minds a bit more? Do our thoughts drift partly because we're not sure that our new activity is important enough – or we're not sure that *we* are very important compared to our children, our husbands, our friends?

And what about the practical demands of housework and childcare – could they be shared more?

Needing to be central

Women grew up with the idea that their home would be their own place, and their special responsibility. They were expected to devote their lives to their families: the only consolation seemed to be that they would be central, the family would rely on them completely. But was that really a good thing for women? (or for their families?) Did it make up for all the self-sacrifice? Were women valued for themselves? or as housekeepers?

For most women, being a housewife was the only thing they thought they could do. Anna Martin, who worked in a working-class women's centre in London around 1911, said that women seemed to *need* their role as mothers; if any change was suggested which meant that women would be less central in the family, the idea caused 'a vague dread'. A generation later, in 1939, the Women's Health Enquiry report said that it was common for a woman to think 'the family could not manage without her'. As the report said, women's involvement with their work in the home was very different from the way most workers felt about their jobs: 'her heart as well as her brains and hands is engaged in her labour.'

So it was hard for women to think of themselves separately from what they did as housewives. Even under impossible conditions most women kept their houses incredibly clean and tidy. As well as being 'their job', it was the only way they had of feeling self-esteem. Women might criticise another woman for 'letting herself go': for example, Margery Spring-Rice, who wrote the Women's Health Enquiry report, was mainly sympathetic to the problems of working-class women. Yet if women chatted to neighbours for a couple of hours, or did *not* keep the house spotless, she remarked on this as if it was a fault.

In 1925, the Women's Co-operative Guild pressed for electricity to be supplied in houses, so that women should have time to do something else in the world besides housework! But as it turned out, electricity was not the answer – housework continued, probably because women lacked the confidence to branch out into new activities.

Could women have arranged to do household tasks together, which might have saved time and energy (and also money)? Sometimes communal facilities were organised, but this was usually in an emergency: for example, in the 1926 miners' strike, there was a communal kitchen in Lochgelly which fed 1,000 people a day very cheaply (at 2d. per head) – the women made most of the food and the men made jam!

Why was this not done more often? Did each woman want to keep her work separate, to show that she was a 'good housewife'? Had women been brought up not to trust each other for help and support?

Occasionally, women were urged to change their attitude. In 1937, an article called 'Where Does Mother Come In?' was published in the *Labour Woman*. The writer said that if husbands and children acted like babies, women had helped to make them so – now they must demand that other members of the family should take more responsibility, otherwise women themselves would be chained down forever.

• Do we still 'need' our responsibilities to our families?

Many women today seem to have a huge sense of responsibility. When in bad situations ourselves, our first thought is often for other people, and we may feel guilty if we cannot provide everything the family seems to need.

A researcher interviewed several pregnant women who were waiting to hear the result of amniocentesis (a test to find out whether their baby might be handicapped). All felt very anxious, but struggled to cope – mainly because they were even more anxious about the effect that their depression might have on the baby.

> 'The first night I couldn't sleep. I lost 4 lb. in weight and kept nearly fainting. . . . I realised that I must pull myself out of it because it wouldn't do the baby any good my being in such a dreadful state.'

> 'I just thought I must eat because the baby must survive.'

Did the women not see themselves as particularly important? Would they have managed to eat for their own sake?

Many women panic when they have to go into hospital for a few days – they plan for neighbours to iron husbands' shirts, and come in and cook. The worry is that husbands and children cannot look after themselves (or maybe that they would resent doing so and think of the woman as 'not a good mother'?). Sometimes women refuse or put off hospital treatment for this reason – putting their own health even more at risk.

Why is it so difficult to share our caring role with other people? A conversation amongst several women showed some of the problems they find about sharing housework:

> 'The thing that men are bad at is doing two things at once, so if I say do you mind looking after Patrick for an hour he'll do it, but you know the washing-up'll still be in the sink when I get back.'

> 'Mine makes a terrible mess – when I was ill there was dust up to here, everything was all over the place. It took me a day to get it all straight.'

> 'So disheartening isn't it.'

> 'He thinks I create work though . . . he says "You're mad, what are you hoovering for, it's not dirty." He doesn't think a thing needs doing unless it's really revolting.'

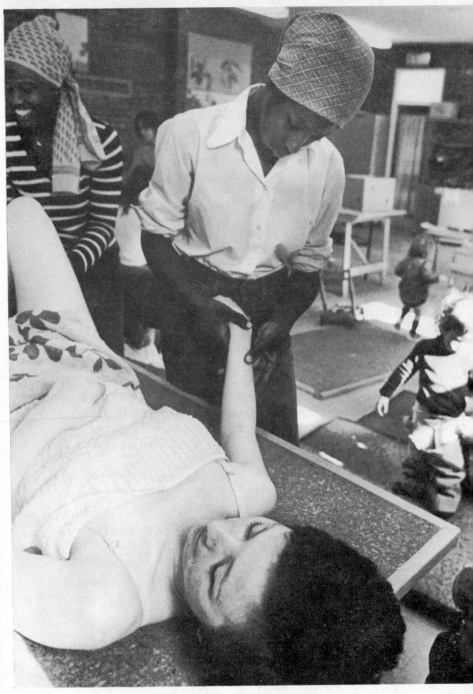

25   Massage class in a Family Centre in Battersea
It is unusual for women to spend time looking after ourselves instead of
looking after others. Can learning about massage and relaxation help us to
feel better?

'I've got to hoover every day because if I don't he does it. That shows me up and makes me feel guilty and I say leave off I'll do it.'

'Oh no I'd let him do it if he wanted to! I'd take pictures as well if he had done.'

This shows how complicated it all is – women worry that men don't care enough, men think that women care too much – and even if men offer to help, it's hard to sit and watch someone else do 'your job' without feeling guilty.

Most men aren't used to looking after people – or looking after houses. How can we get them more used to doing this? And why do women have such high standards? Why can't we feel comfortable if our houses or our children are untidy sometimes? Could we try to separate ourselves off from it all a bit more?

Even women in paid jobs often worry about doing well enough; especially in caring jobs which are like our work at home, we tend to be conscientious to a point way beyond what is necessary, sometimes driving ourselves to illness through the strain.

Do we tend to make matters worse by criticising ourselves *and* other women for not doing well enough? In the conversation reported above, women also said:

'I think psychologically you need to have a tidy house.'

'You probably do it yourself, if you walk into someone's house and it's chaos you do think "oh, she doesn't care".'

The pressures to be the perfect housewife and mother seem to come from within ourselves, as well as from advertisements and from the men around us. Even when there are no men around, within a group of women, we can reinforce each other's feelings of responsibility and we can lack self-confidence. All our upbringing has prepared us to doubt whether we have a personality other than the role of wife or mother.

Keeping quiet

Drug companies want us to take pills so that we don't notice our problems any more. Other companies also offer us products which they say will help us to cope – Yeast-Vite for extra energy; Radox baths so that you are calm and refreshed when your husband comes home, and you don't bother him by being tense and upset after being with the children all day.

In other words, we are not supposed to talk about our real lives to anyone – we should carry on uncomplainingly.

Maybe some illnesses come from keeping quiet. Why do so many women get migraines, or pre-menstrual tension? Does this sometimes happen instead of being angry about our situation? Is illness any answer? Could we start to change things?

What some women have done

Many women have stood up for themselves with courage in their everyday lives – it was something they decided to do on their own. Some have had long battles with welfare officials:

'Finally the drains blocked completely on a Sunday and I had to pay to have it done – but I kept all the receipts and I went on and on at the Housing Office till I got the money back and £20 compensation.'

'I'd been waiting to be re-housed for a year. It was impossible to live in that flat, being in a wheelchair. Finally I got all my belongings packed into a van, and a friend drove me to the Housing Office. I got out my sleeping bag and everything and said "Right, from now on I'm living here until you find me somewhere decent." Within a few hours they'd come up with that "impossible to get" ground-floor flat.'

Other women have asserted themselves with doctors:

'I get them to explain it to me, I want a copy of what they've written down.'

'That room they use at . . . hospital [for child development tests] well it frightened me, and Jane had had her hearing test done at the clinic and this was just for their research . . . they asked me to bring her back again so I said I wouldn't do it, I said look this place frightens me so can you imagine how a child of a year and a half feels.'

The hardest place to make changes is often within the family. But sometimes the last straw comes after years of pressure:

'My son, he came in last night and said where's my dinner. I

said don't treat me like that, I've given up a lot for you, and now you're acting just like your father. . . . I told him to cook his own dinner.'

What can you do when a man won't get up in the night for the children?

'Mine just wakes up and moans.'

'Well I kicked mine out of bed last night.'

'I stick the baby on top of him, crying and everything, while I get her feed ready.'

Do you always have to cook?

'The first Sunday after we married I stayed in bed and he had to cook. I bet he thought "I've got a right one here." But he's done it ever since.'

'His friends used to all happen to come round at dinnertime . . . now I just sit down and eat my meal, I tell him, if you want them to eat, give it to them off your own plate.'

How can you get men to realise what it's like being stuck at home?

'He had the kids for about four days when I was ill and he said I know what it's like now, it must drive you mad because you have to do everything, housework, shopping, kids.'

'When he's going to go out I turn round and say, if I can't go out you're not going out and he knows I mean it, so he's getting a bit better now, he lets me out now and again.'

'I hand him the baby and say "I'm just going out for a minute" . . . and I turn it into four hours.'

'When he comes back in the middle of the night I lock him out and pretend to be asleep.'

Can your children help you?

'I want my children to be really independent. I think they can help me too . . . my three year old, when she wants a snack she makes herself a peanut butter sandwich.'

What can you do if your husband is expecting you to 'manage' with money?

'He was giving me hardly any housekeeping money. So I bought

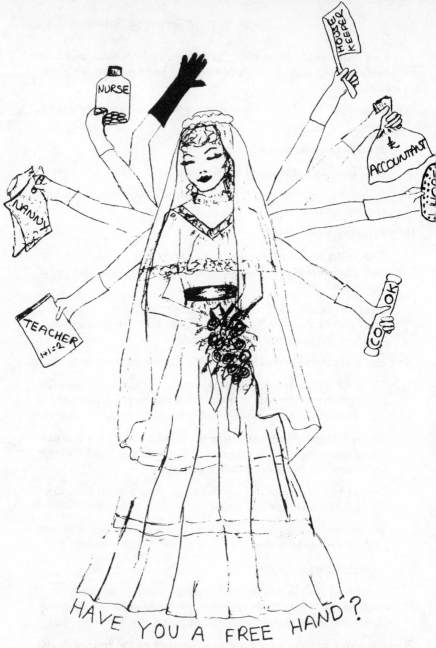

NURSE

HOUSE KEEPER

NANNY

ACCOUNTANT £

TEACHER 1+1=2

COOK

HAVE YOU A FREE HAND?

26 'Have You A Free Hand?': illustration for a pamphlet on marriage by
women from the Lambeth Health Bus
Anne drew this picture to show the many responsibilities which marriage
often brings for women. In the pamphlet she writes, 'I had hoped I would be
the lucky one and that marriage would be different for me . . . four years
and two children later, his attitudes haven't changed and I am constantly
fighting them.' Can marriage be different?

*food for me and the children and none for him. When he
complained I said what do you expect? Then he gave me more.
And he never did it again.'*

*'I got so fed up, I threw him out, and I only had him back on the
condition he gives me all his wages and I give him £25 back.'*

Alternative ways of living

Some women find that the man they live with will share the work
at home. But many women today decide to live alone, or by themselves with their children, rather than live with a man who expects
constant services but gives little in return. As one woman summed
it up: 'I do a lot less work now he's living somewhere else.'

A woman who escaped from her violent husband to the safety
of a Women's Aid refuge commented

*'You want to get a bit of peace. You get so used to being
domineered, it feels like heaven, being here. In a way, this is
more normal living than some women have at home, mentally
wise. You live your life, you do what you want. You've got more
freedom.'*

Being on our own is a situation which most women have not
been brought up to expect. It can be hard in some ways, rewarding
in others.

*'I was worried I'd be lonely without him. I do worry about being
alone in the house, I get nervous about someone breaking in.
But other than that, I don't miss him at all.'*

'It's so nice on my own. I just sit and do my knitting in peace.'
(women talking about separating from their husbands)

Living alone *can* mean loneliness and extra responsibility –
especially if you have children. Some women decide to live in a
household with other people – maybe these will be other women,
maybe they will include men as well, maybe there will be several
parents with children. In these households, people usually take it
in turns to do the cleaning and cooking, and everyone helps to look
after the children.

*'I'd like to find somewhere more caring. I'd like to be with other
people who'd be company and they'd help me out. It's such a*

worry being by myself – who's going to look after the children when I'm ill?' (a woman looking for a collective household to live in)

Are there different alternatives for women now? Can we arrange our lives so that we have satisfying, close relationships with others, which involve mutual support?

New feelings about sexuality

Another place where we may be able to make changes is in our feelings about sexuality. This often seems a private subject, the hardest thing of all to discuss with other people. Yet women are beginning to talk about this together and to decide, each for ourselves, how we would like things to be different.

There can be much more to sexuality than sexual relationships alone. Many women think that it is important to feel happy and relaxed about ourselves, which may mean, again, making *time* somehow. One women's group agreed that each person would do something special for herself before the next meeting. They reported later:

'I spent a whole hour in the bath yesterday. I filled it right up to the top – it was the first time I'd ever allowed myself more than a few inches of water. It was lovely, just lying there.'

'I bought myself two records and a bunch of roses. I felt great!'

Sharing warmth and affection with other people is also a basic need in our lives. Often emotional closeness with women friends is particularly important.

'It's so nice being in a group with women – we tell each other quite personal things. We all went away for a weekend – just women – and we had such a good laugh.' (woman in a health group)

Can sexual relationships follow freer paths than the patterns we have been brought up in? Relationships between women may be based on a more equal exchange of affection and a more relaxed view of sex.

'With my girlfriend there was no beginning and no end when we made love. Sometimes she had an orgasm, or I did – that

was just one of the things that could happen along the way.'
(from the book *For Ourselves*)

Many women are determined to try to make sexual relationships with men different too.

'With my present lover I made sure it was completely different right from the start. We asked each other what we liked . . . we started very carefully, step by step. . . . We can be tender with each other . . . if he caresses me very softly on my hair, I get such a rare feeling.' (from *For Ourselves*)

Feeling more at home with our own bodies, and enjoying different kinds of relationships with the people we are close to, is part of the new strength which women are starting to gain.

Confidence and health

Every small action is important, because it means self-respect and confidence. Our mental health certainly improves if we are feeling stronger in situations. Probably our physical health does too. Health means total well-being – we can become healthier in many different ways. For example, by getting involved in a women's health group, a woman might gain more confidence in herself – even though she might not immediately make changes like giving up smoking. Overall, her well-being would be increasing step by step. Often, once changes start, there is no going back.

'This is community education for you – it's given me something – believe it or not, I couldn't speak to nobody before, but now I'll fight anybody, for my kids especially.' (woman explaining how she felt about a health course)

'When you come somewhere like this you become a person, you're you . . . now I've done this I'd find it very hard just to go back.' (woman from Save Bethnal Green Hospital Campaign)

Or, as a woman wrote many years ago when she went to her first meeting of the Women's Co-operative Guild: 'I had longings and aspirations and a vague idea of power within myself which had never had an opportunity for realisation.' Can we find this power too?

CONCLUSION

Has women's health improved since the 1930s?

Although living conditions are mostly better now, many people still have to face poverty and bad housing, while others live in comparative luxury. And there are new and different threats to our health – more isolation for women at home, pressures to slim, dangerous contraceptives, chemical hazards. . . .

Maybe we can't measure 'improvements'. We can only say that our health problems are in some ways different. But the same areas remain important – for example, work, food, housing, contraception and abortion. If our health is to improve, we are talking about having more control over community services, over working conditions, over the food we can buy, over the environment we live in, over the way money is distributed. . . . We are also talking about challenging the way *caring* is organised – housework, childcare, keeping people going.

Caring is vitally needed – but if one person is looking after a child or a sick elderly parent alone, trying to satisfy their needs day and night, that person's life is taken over and their health suffers. If the work is shared, it gives some freedom and independence (and better health) to everyone who joins in.

Women are constantly giving out practical and emotional support, and getting very little back. Even a woman without children finds that there are always men to be mothered, after all. Other people make the most of the caring – yet sometimes they resent it too, they feel overwhelmed by it. Do women perhaps 'overdo the caring' in ways which are not good for ourselves or other people? Is it helpful never to say 'No'? – always to be self-sacrificing? Can we develop new ways of caring – a balance between giving to other people and answering our own needs? Would this help everyone to be more independent and build up the strength to lead their own lives?

It certainly seems that it would help women. We need to put

some caring into ourselves for a change. If we always cope, the system never shows any cracks. We crack up instead.

We need to believe we are important, that we deserve to be treated equally and we deserve better health. Seeing ourselves as independent people is the first step. I began writing this book determined not to call women 'wives' or 'mothers'. Often I found myself doing so automatically. It was amazing how crossing out 'wives' and 'mothers', and writing 'women' instead, gave a completely different feeling – of people in our own right, individuals with the ability to actively change our lives.

We are taking on powerful forces, but we also have immense potential. Through small steps or large ones, we can work towards becoming healthier and more confident. We can begin to speak out and share our experiences, to decide what we want to change and act on it. We can begin to make 'time for ourselves'.

USEFUL INFORMATION

Joining a women's group – or setting one up

A women's health group may form with a particular interest: for example, food and eating, or depression. Other groups may decide to look at a wide range of issues. Groups can often provide an alternative to going as an individual to see a doctor: some women may want to do both. Suggested activities for women's health groups are listed at the end of each chapter in this book.

To meet other women locally, and find out about health groups and health courses: check for advertisements on notice-boards in health centres and community centres. To help start a group, you could advertise in shop windows or write a letter to the local paper. A group could also begin with friends meeting in each other's houses.

The following central places could help you to find local contacts:

WIRES P.O. Box 162, Sheffield 1 1UD (0742-755290), national information service and newsletter for the women's liberation movement (knows of local women's centres and women's groups).

Spare Rib 27 Clerkenwell Close, London EC1, a monthly women's liberation magazine (carries advertisements for local groups needing new members).

Pre-School Playgroups Association Alford House, Aveline St, London SE11 (01-582 8871).

Gingerbread (self-help association for single parents) 35 Wellington St, London WC2 (01-240 0953/4).

Ask your Community Health Council, or your Adult Education Institute or branch of the Workers' Educational Association (WEA) if they are running a health course – or could plan one for the future. Adult education institutes often have a community education section which might fund a special course for your group.

Community Health Council (CHC) Look in the phone book, or Yellow Pages or local directory, under Community Health Councils or Health.

Adult education Look in Yellow Pages or local directory, under Education.

WEA Central contact is: 9 Upper Berkeley St, London W1 (01-402 5608) or in Manchester (061-325 9972).

CHCs should know about groups working on health issues too. Your tenants' group may be campaigning about health and housing. Trade unions run courses on health and safety at work, and women's issues – check with your shop steward or safety representative. Maybe you yourself could become a shop steward or safety rep?

Note on using the quizzes

Writing quizzes like the ones in this book and doing them as a group could be a good way to get a discussion going. One method is for everyone to answer the first question, then fold back that question and pass the paper on to the next person: then answer the next question, and so on. This keeps the answers anonymous, which some people may prefer. When the quiz is finished, you can find out the general feeling of the group by taking each question in turn and looking at how many people answered (a), (b), (c) or (d). During the discussion, people will be able to talk about their own answers if they wish.

Contacts list

These organisations may know of local groups – please write and ask (with a stamped addressed envelope!). Note: each year, *Spare Rib* (see 'Joining a women's group') produces a diary with a comprehensive list of contacts useful to women.

• Black women

OWAAD (*Organisation of Women of Asian and African Descent*) c/o Black Women's Centre, 41 Stockwell Green, London SW9 (01-274 9220).

Black Health Workers' and Patients' Group 146 Kentish Town Rd, London NW1.

Sickle Cell Society c/o Brent Community Health Council, 16 High St, London NW10 4LX (01-451 3293).

• Cancer

Women's National Cancer Control Campaign 1 South Audley St, London W1 (01-499 7532).

• Caring

Association of Carers 58 New Rd, Chatham, Kent (Medway 813981).

• Contraception and abortion

Brook Advisory Centres (especially for young people) 153a East St, London SE17 (01-708 1234/1390).

FPIS (*Family Planning Information Service*) 27–35 Mortimer St, London W1 (01-636 7866).

NAC (*National Abortion Campaign*) 374 Gray's Inn Rd, London WC1 (01-278 0153).

• Women with disabilities

Sisters Against Disablement c/o Lesley Wilde, 2 Mereworth Drive, London SE18 (01-854 6561).

Liberation Network of People with Disabilities c/o Flat 4, 188 Ramsden Rd, London SW12 (01-673 4310).

• Drugs, alcohol, smoking

Release (drugs) 1 Elgin Ave, London W9 (01-289 1123).

DAWN (*Drugs Alcohol and Women Nationally*) c/o London Council on Alcoholism, 146 Victoria St, London EC4.

ASH (*Action on Smoking and Health*) 27–35 Mortimer St, London W1 (01-637 9843).

• Environment

CLEAR (*Campaign for Lead-Free Air*) 2 Northdown St, London N1.

Friends of the Earth 377 City Rd, London EC1 (01-833 0731).

• Health information (general)

Women's Health Information Centre Ufton Community Centre, 12 Ufton Rd, London N1 5BY (01-254 9094).

Politics of Health Group c/o 9 Poland St, London W1 (has groups which work on specific issues, e.g. food, alternative medicine).

Spare Rib magazine (see p. 151) and **Outwrite** women's newspaper, Oxford House, Derbyshire St, London E2, often carry articles on health. **Spare Rib** has a checklist of articles from previous issues.

See Red Poster Collective 16a Iliffe Yard, off Crampton St, London SE17 (01-701 8314) – posters on women's lives, and health topics.

Health Education Council 78 New Oxford St, London WC1 (01-637 1881).

• Health service rights

Your local **Community Health Council** (see 'Joining a women's group') and **CHC News** 363 Euston Rd, London NW1 (01-388 4943).

Maternity Alliance 309 Kentish Town Rd, London NW5 (01-267 3255).

• Health workers

Association of Radical Midwives c/o 8a The Drive, Wimbledon, London SW20.

Radical Nurses' Group 20 Melrose Rd, Sheffield 3, or c/o 9 Ryland Rd, London NW5.

Radical Health Visitors' Group c/o BSSRS, 9 Poland St, London W1.

Women in Medicine c/o 10 Sotheby Rd, London N5 (01-226 3441).

● **Housing**

SCAT (*Services to Community Action and Tenants*) 31 Clerkenwell Close, London EC1 (01-253 3627).

● **Lesbians**

Lesbian Line BM Box 1514, London WC1N 3XX (01-837 8602).

● **Therapy**

Women's Therapy Centre 6 Manor Gardens, London N7 (01-263 6200).

● **Violence against women**

Women's Aid Federation 374 Gray's Inn Rd, London WC1 (01-837 9316).

Rape Crisis Centre P.O. Box 69, London WC1X 9NJ (01-837 1600, 24-hour line).

● **Welfare rights/women's rights**

Citizens' Advice Bureaux (CABs) 110 Drury Lane, London WC2 (01-836 9231) or in local phone book.

Law Centres Federation 164 North Gower St, London NW1 (01-387 8570) to find local law centres.

One-Parent Families 255 Kentish Town Rd, London NW5 (01-267 1361).

Claimants' Union Federation Bethnal Green Rights Shop, 296 Bethnal Green Rd, London E2 (01-739 4173).

Rights of Women 374 Gray's Inn Rd, London WC1 (01-278 6349).

EOC (*Equal Opportunities Commission*) Overseas House, Quay St, Manchester 3 (061-833 9244).

- **Work (paid)**

Hazards Group and **Women and Work Hazards Group** c/o BSSRS, 9 Poland St, London W1.

London Homeworking Campaign 10 Burnays Grove, London SW9.

Low Pay Unit 9 Poland St, London W1 (01-437 1780).

Women's Campaign for Jobs 165 Liverpool Rd, London N1 (01-278 1341).

- **Young women**

NAYC (*National Association of Youth Clubs*) **Girls' Work** 30 Peacock Lane, Leicester LE1 5NY (0533–29514).

Health booklist

To find your nearest bookshop with a good range of women's books, write for the *Radical Bookshop Guide*, 60p from Federation of Radical Booksellers, c/o Oakleaf Books, 109 Church St, Milton Keynes.

- **General books on women's lives**

Women in the 80's (Counter Information Service, 9 Poland St, London W1, 1981, 95p): survey of our current situation: looks at work, the law, violence against women, etc.

Housewife Ann Oakley (Pelican, Harmondsworth, 1982, £1.95): contains interviews in which women describe their lives.

As Things Are: Women, work and family in South London (Bonfire Press, Union Place Resource Centre, 122–124 Vassall Rd, London SW9 6JB, 1976, 50p plus postage): interviews with women about low-paid work, and housing action.

Women in Collective Action (Association of Community Workers, 22 Colombo St, London SE1 8DP, 1982, £4.95): women's groups describe action in their local neighbourhoods.

• General books on health and health services

It's My Life, Doctor (Brent Community Health Council, 16 High St, London NW10, 1981, free to people living in Brent, 65p incl. p&p to others): looks at seven common health problems including bronchitis and depression, their causes, and what could be done about them.

Women's Health and . . . Unemployment, Food, Smoking, History, Work and Stress (Women's Health Information Centre, Ufton Community Centre, Ufton Rd, London N1, 10p each plus S.A.E.): series of leaflets.

The Political Economy of Health Lesley Doyal with Imogen Pennell (Pluto, London, 1979, £4.95): discusses how the organisation of society (in Britain and internationally) affects health.

The Black Report on Inequalities in Health DHSS (DHSS Leaflets Unit, Canons Park, Government Buildings, Honeypot Lane, Stanmore, Middx, 1980, £8 plus 50p p&p): results of a major survey on ill-health in Britain.

• Alcohol

Women Under the Influence Brigid McConville (Virago, London, 1983, £3.50): why women have drinking problems and what you can do about them.

• A woman's body

Our Bodies Ourselves Angela Phillips and Jill Rakusen, eds (Penguin, Harmondsworth, 1979, £4.50): handbook on our female biology, contraception, sexuality and many other topics.

Down There (Onlywomen Press, London, 1980, 75p): explains how to do self-examination.

• Alternative medicine

Alternative Medicine Andrew Stanway (Pelican, Harmondsworth, 1982, £2.95): guide to alternative therapies.

The Massage Book George Downing (Penguin, Harmondsworth, 1982, £1.95): explains simple massage techniques.

- **Black women**

Black People and the Health Service (Brent Community Health Council, 16 High St, London NW10, 1981, free to people living in Brent, 65p incl. p&p to others): report on racism in the NHS.

Asian Women Speak Out (National Extension College, 18 Brooklands Ave, Cambridge CB2 2HN, 1980, £1): an illustrated reader with quotes from Asian women about their lives.

Finding a Voice Amrit Wilson (Virago, London, 1981, £3.50): looks at Asian women's experiences in Britain.

- **Childbirth**

Every Birth it comes Different Hackney Reading Centre (Centerprise, 136 Kingsland High St, London E8, 1980, £1.20): women describe their experiences of childbirth.

Your Body, Your Baby, Your Life Angela Phillips (Pandora Press, London, 1983, £3.95): guide to pregnancy, birth and caring for your baby.

The Short Report (HMSO, P.O. Box 569, London SE1 9NH, 1980, £5): investigation into the causes of infant death and handicap in Britain – discusses the NHS facilities provided for pregnancy and childbirth.

- **Cystitis**

Cystitis: A Complete Self-Help Guide Angela Kilmartin (Hamlyn, Feltham, 1981, £1): simple instructions for avoiding cystitis attacks.

- **Women with disabilities**

Better Lives for Disabled Women Jo Campling (Virago, London, 1979, £1.25): short sections on relationships, sexuality, menstruation, rights to benefits, etc.

Images of Ourselves ed. Jo Campling (Routledge & Kegan Paul, London, 1981, £3.95): women with different disabilities write about their lives.

● Fertility control

Safe Sex and *A Look at Safe Sex* (Brook Advisory Centres Education and Publications Unit, 10 Albert St, Birmingham B4 7UD, 1979, 20p each plus 25p for p&p): leaflets on contraception. The first is detailed, the second contains drawings showing how to use the different methods.

Abortion: Our Struggle for Control (National Abortion Campaign, 374 Gray's Inn Rd, London WC1, 25p plus postage): short articles on women's right to safe, legal abortion facilities.

Mixed Feelings (Brent Against Corrie Group, 1980, 30p plus postage from NAC as above): ten women talk about their experiences of unplanned pregnancy, and abortion.

The Experience of Infertility Naomi Pfeffer and Anne Woollett (Virago, London, 1983, £3.50): feelings about infertility, and practical information about the possible solutions.

● Food and nutrition

Food and Profit (Politics of Health Group, c/o BSSRS, 9 Poland St, London W1, 50p plus 20p for p&p): explains how the food we eat can harm our health.

Who Really Starves? Lisa Leghorn and Mary Roodowsky (Friendship Press, 1977, £1.95 from Third World Publications, 151 Stratford Rd, Birmingham B11 1RD): looks at how women all over the world lack good food.

Fat is a Feminist Issue Susie Orbach (Hamlyn, Feltham, 1983, £1.50): discusses why women have eating problems, and how to give up dieting.

Prevention of Handicap and the Health of Women Margaret and Arthur Wynn (Routledge & Kegan Paul, 1979, £10.75): argues that lack of good food affects women's health and the health of their babies.

● Housing

Campaigning Against Dampness (Services to Community Action and Tenants, 31 Clerkenwell Close, London EC1, 60p incl. p&p to tenants and trade union organisations, £1 incl. p&p to others): practical suggestions for what tenants can do about damp housing.

● Menopause

Menopause: A Positive Approach Rosetta Reitz (Allen & Unwin, 1981, £2.95): looks at the difficulties and the rewarding times women have experienced during menopause.

● Mental health

Trouble With Tranquillisers (Release Publications, 1 Elgin Ave, London W9, 1982, 40p plus p&p): practical suggestions for getting off tranquillisers.

Postnatal Depression Vivienne Welburn (Fontana, London, 1980, £1.25): includes interviews with women who have experienced this.

In Our Own Hands Sheila Ernst and Lucy Goodison (Women's Press, London, 1981, £4.50): guide to self-help therapy.

● Periods

Why Suffer?: Periods and their Problems Lynda Birke and Katy Gardner (Virago, London, 1982, £2.50): explanation of menstrual cycle, ideas to help with period pains.

● Sexuality

For Ourselves Anja Meulenbelt (Sheba, London, 1981, £4.50): looks at how we can create a new, positive attitude towards women's sexuality.

We're Here Angela Stewart-Park and Jules Cassidy (Quartet, London, 1977, £1.95): interviews with lesbian women.

The Hite Report Shere Hite (Dell, New York, 1981, £3.50): results of a detailed survey on women's sexuality.

● Smoking

The Ladykillers Bobbie Jacobson (Pluto, London, 1981, £1.95): how cigarette companies persuade women to smoke – and how to give up.

• Violence against women

Clout!: The Story Behind the Bruises (Commonword, 61 Bloom St, Manchester, 1979, 50p): interviews with women at a Women's Aid Refuge.

Battered Women and the New Law Anna Coote and Tess Gill (InterAction and NCCL, London, 1979, 85p): practical guide.

Stand Your Ground Kaleghl Quinn (Orbis, London, 1983, £3.95): guide to self-defence for women.

• Welfare rights

Behind Closed Doors Equal Opportunities Commission (EOC, Overseas House, Quay St, Manchester 3, 1981, free): survey on careers.

Women's Rights: A Practical Guide Anna Coote and Tess Gill (Penguin, Harmondsworth, 1981, £3.95): explains the law.

Women and the Welfare State Elizabeth Wilson (Tavistock, London, 1977, £3.95): how the Welfare State has affected women, in the past and today.

The following have many publications, especially leaflets and pamphlets; write for details:

National Council for Civil Liberties (NCCL), 21 Tabard St, London SE1 (01-403 3888).

Child Poverty Action Group, 1 Macklin St, Drury Lane, London WC2 (01-242 9149/3225).

• Working conditions

The Hazards Group, and Women and Work Hazards Group, c/o BSSRS, 9 Poland St, London W1, have a large publications list, including:

Danger: Women At Work (Women and Work Hazards Group, 1983): pamphlet explaining common hazards and the rights of safety representatives.

Office Workers' Survival Handbook Marianne Craig (BSSRS, 1981, £2.70 plus 30p p&p): comprehensive guide to office safety.

History booklist

Working-Class Wives: Their Health and Conditions Margery Spring-Rice (republished Virago, London, 1981, £2.95): report of the Women's Health Enquiry survey of the late 1930s.

Maternity: Letters from Working Women ed. Margaret Llewelyn Davies (republished Virago, London, 1978, £2.95): collection of letters to the Women's Co-operative Guild in 1914.

Round About a Pound a Week Maud Pember Reeves (republished Virago, London, 1982, £3.50): women's budgets early in this century.

The Hard Way Up Hannah Mitchell (republished Virago, London, 1977, £2.95): autobiography of a campaigner for women's rights and socialism.

The Tamarisk Tree: Vol. I Dora Russell (Virago, London, 1980, £3.50): describes the struggle to make birth control available in the 1920s.

A New World for Women: Stella Browne, Socialist Feminist Sheila Rowbotham (Pluto, London, 1977, £1.95): the ideas of a woman who campaigned for abortion rights in the 1930s.

The Politics of Motherhood: Child and Maternal Welfare in England 1900–39 Jane Lewis (Croom Helm, London, 1980, £10.95): detailed survey of this period.

Hidden From History Sheila Rowbotham (Pluto, London, 1983, £2.95): introduction to women's history.

Witches, Midwives and Nurses and *Complaints and Disorders* Barbara Ehrenreich and Deirdre English (Writers and Readers, London, 1973, 65p and 85p): the first is a history of women as healers, the second looks at how 'women's illnesses' have been seen in the past.

Finding out about women's history

You could start by talking to older women (relatives, friends, members of local women's organisations): maybe you could tape discussions with them and make a pamphlet about women's experiences in the past.

Your library may have a local history section, with someone to advise you. They may also keep old newspapers. Ask at local museums too.

Ask for an adult education class on women's history from your local Adult Education Institute or branch of the Workers' Educational Association (WEA) – maybe you could help to set the course up?

Discovering Women's History: A Practical Manual by Deirdre Beddoe (Pandora Press, London, 1983, £3.95) gives lots of suggestions for starting on local history projects, with lists of useful libraries, and local women's history groups.

Places which I found particularly useful when preparing this book were:

The Fawcett Library, City of London Polytechnic, Old Castle St, London E1 7NT (01-283 1030 x570): a special library for women's history, full of pamphlets, books, pictures and newspaper cuttings from centuries ago to the present day. (Thanks especially to David Doughan for helping me to find material.)

British Library Newspaper Section, Colindale Avenue, London NW9 (01-200 5515): has copies of old newspapers and magazines. See especially *Labour Woman, Woman's Dreadnought, Woman Worker, Out of Work, Unemployed Worker.*

National Museum of Labour History, Limehouse Town Hall, Commercial Rd, London E14 (01-515 3229): has a collection of labour movement documents and photographs. (Thanks to Jane Roberts for her help.)

Labour Party Library, 150 Walworth Rd, London SE17 1JT (01-703 0833): has copies of *Labour Woman* newspaper and a photograph collection. (Thanks to Ursula Alexis and Ruby Ranaweera for their help.)

Manchester Studies Archive of Family Photographs, Manchester Polytechnic, Cavendish House, Cavendish St, Manchester M15 6BG (061-228 6171 x2551): large collection of historical photographs.

The Feminist Library and Information Centre, Hungerford House, Victoria Embankment, London WC2 (01-930 0715) has a library of books about women and acts as a point of contact for women interested in doing any kind of research.

The historical part of *No Time For Women* is based on my thesis: *The Politics of Married Working-Class Women's Health*

Care in Britain, 1918–1939 (Charmian Kenner, M.Phil. in History and Social Studies of Science, University of Sussex, 1979). This contains a lot of detailed information and a long booklist. You can obtain a microfilm of the thesis by asking your nearest central library to get it from the British Library Lending Division, Boston Spa, and giving the following identification number: D40643/82. There are also copies of the thesis in the University of Sussex Library (numbered S1599), the Fawcett Library and the Feminist Library and Information Centre (as above).

Sources for this book

Sources for the quotes and information in *No Time For Women* include:

Alison Macfarlane, 'Birth, Death and Handicap; saving money, spending lives', *Science for People* 48, Spring 1981.

Sylvia Shimmin, Joyce McNally, Sonia Liff, 'Pressures on women engaged in factory work', *Employment Gazette*, August 1981.

Penny Mansfield, 'With stars in their eyes and a wife at the sink', *Guardian*, 9 February 1982.

National Abortion Campaign, *Abortion Internationally* and *Abortion – The Evidence: A Report from the Tribunal on Abortion Rights, January 1977*.

Keith Armstrong and Huw Beynon, eds, *Hello, Are You Working? Memories of the Thirties in the North East of England* (Strong Words Press, Whitley Bay, 1977).

'GP's report from the front line on jobless casualties', *Guardian*, 24 August 1981.

Jeanne Stellman, *Women's Work, Women's Health* (Pantheon Books, London, 1977).

Gail Barlow, 'Midwifery in Manchester in the 1930's', unpublished paper.

Elizabeth Wilson, 'Who really gets the benefit from this sort of self-sacrifice', *Guardian*, 7 January 1982.

Family Group, Peckham Health Project, *Scream* (pamphlet).

'My world became the size of my baby', *Spare Rib* 47, June 1976.

'Netherley United: women take on the housing corporation', *Spare Rib* 56, March 1977.

'High Rise, High Rent', *Spare Rib* 41, December 1975.

'We grow wise through it: the EGA hospital occupation', *Spare Rib* 55, February 1977.

'Save the Green: Bethnal Green Hospital occupation', *Spare Rib* 77, December 1978.

'A Cost Counted in Lives', *Women's Voice*, no. 7.

'Women Cleaners Fight Asbestos Dust', *Hazards Bulletin* 5, December 1976.

'Tenants Fight Killer Asbestos', *Hazards Bulletin* 20, March 1980.

Sources also include the following books, details of which appear in the booklists:

Working-Class Wives, Maternity: Letters from Working Women, Finding A Voice, Prevention of Handicap and the Health of Women, Clout, Behind Closed Doors, Black People and the Health Service, For Ourselves, Food and Profit, Women in the 80's, Women in Collective Action (article 'Coming Alive Hurts' by South Wales Tenants' Association), *Mixed Feelings, As Things Are.*

There are full references to the historical material in *The Politics of Married Working-Class Women's Health Care in Britain, 1918–39*: see 'Finding out about women's history' section.

INDEX

PANDORA PRESS

an imprint of Routledge and Kegan Paul

ELIZABETH GASKELL : FOUR SHORT STORIES

The Three Eras of Libbie Marsh · Lizzie Leigh · The Well of Pen-Morfa · The Manchester Marriage

In her unaffected, direct description of the lives of working class women as lived out between the mean streets and the cotton mills of nineteenth century England, Elizabeth Gaskell chose to break with the literary conventions of Victorian ladies' fiction (which demanded genteel romances) and give her readers, instead, the harsh realities, the defiance and courage those lives entailed. Far from being delicate drawing room flowers, the characters in these four stories (collected here for the first time) are women who live unsupported by men, who labour and love and scheme and survive in strangely modern tales shot through with Gaskell's integrity of observation and deep compassion. The stories are prefaced by a long appreciation of Gaskell's life and work by Anna Walters.

'Mrs Gaskell draws the distinction between male and female values quietly, but forcefully' *School Librarian*

0-86358-001-7 Fiction/Criticism 122pp 198 × 129 mm introduced by Anna Walters paperback.

ALL THE BRAVE PROMISES

Memories of Aircraftwomen 2nd Class 2146391

Mary Lee Settle

Mary Lee Settle was a young American woman living a comfortable life in Washington D.C. when the Second World War broke out. In 1942 she boarded a train, carrying 'a last bottle of champagne and an armful of roses', and left for England to join the WAAF. She witnessed the horror of war – the bombing raids, the planes lost in fog, the children evacuated, a blacked-out Britain of austerity and strain. She also witnessed the women, her fellow recruits, as they struggled to adapt to their new identities and new lives at the bottom of the uniformed pile. Dedicated 'to the wartime other ranks of the Women's Auxiliary Air Force – below the rank of Sergeant', this rare book captures women's wartime experience; a remarkable and important story by one of America's prizewinning novelists.

'One of the most moving accounts of war experience ever encountered' *Library Journal*

0-86358-033-5 General/Autobiography 160pp 198 × 129 mm paperback

not for sale in the U.S.A. or Canada

MY COUNTRY IS THE WHOLE WORLD

an anthology of women's work on peace and war

Cambridge Women's Peace Collective (eds)

Women's struggle for peace is no recent phenomenon. In this book, the work of women for peace from 600 BC to the present is documented in a unique collection of extracts from songs, poems, diaries, letters, petitions, pictures, photographs and pamphlets through the ages. A book to give as a gift, to read aloud from, to research from, to teach from, *My Country is the Whole World* is both a resource and an inspiration for all who work for peace today.

'an historic document . . . readers will be amazed at the extent of the collection' *Labour Herald*

'a beautifully presented and illustrated book which makes for accessible and enlightening reading' *Morning Star*

0-86358-004-1 Social Questions/History 306pp A5 illustrated throughout paperback

DISCOVERING WOMEN'S HISTORY

a practical manual

Deirdre Beddoe

Rainy Sunday afternoons, long winter evenings: why not set yourself a research project, either on your own or in a group or classroom? This is the message from Deirdre Beddoe, an historian who tears away the mystique of her own profession in this step-by-step guide to researching the lives of ordinary women in Britain from 1800 to 1945. *Discovering Women's History* tells you how to get started on the detective trail of history and how to stalk your quarry through attics and art galleries, museums and old newspapers, church archives and the Public Records Office – and how to publish your findings once you have completed your project.

'an invaluable and fascinating guide to the raw material for anyone approaching this unexplored territory' *The Sunday Times*

'Thrilling and rewarding and jolly good fun' *South Wales Argus*

0-86358-008-4 Hobbies/Social History 232pp 198 × 129 mm illustrated